Basic Principles
of Robotic Mastectomy
and Immediate
Breast Reconstruction

Hyung Seok Park MD, PhD

Associate Professor
Department of Surgery, Yonsei University College of Medicine
Breast Cancer Center, Yonsei Cancer Center
Yonsei University Health System, Seoul, Korea

Basic Principles of Robotic Mastectomy and Immediate Breast Reconstruction

1st Edition Printed | July 9, 2021
1st Edition Issued | July 23, 2021

Edited by	Hyung Seok Park
Planned by	Andy Lim
Publisher	Ju-Yeun Chang
Editing Design by	Eun-Jung Yang
Cover Design by	Jae-Wook Kim
Illustrated by	Ho-Hyeon Lee
Produced by	Soon-Ho Lee
Publishing House	Koonja Publishing, Inc.

Registration No. 4-139 (June 24, 1991)
Paju Publishing Complex, 338, Hoedong-gil (474-1 Seopae-dong),
Paju-si, Gyeonggi-do, South Korea (10881)
Telephone: (031) 943-1888 Fax: (031) 955-9545
Website: www.koonja.co.kr

ISBN 979-11-5955-730-9

Basic Principles of Robotic Mastectomy and Immediate Breast Reconstruction

When I was a child, robots seemed to be a kind of fantasy. Controlling huge robot machines that resemble movement of humans, like in the famous animations 'Gundam' and 'Mazinger Z', fascinated a little kid's mind. Even though the actual technical progress of robot systems is not the same as that in the fantasy of my childhood, robots have changed a lot of things in our lives. Many automated robot systems are used in many different industries. They make a huge number of products from delicate and complex semi-conductors to heavy machines such as cars and air-planes. The surgical field also is being revolutionized.

Nowadays, robotic surgical systems have changed surgeons' experience. Endoscopic or laparoscopic surgery can provide minimally invasive surgery for patients. There is no difference between endoscopic and robotic surgery in terms of the patients' outcomes. However, robotic surgery definitely delivers a better experience for surgeons than endoscopic surgery.

Robotic breast surgery was first introduced by several pioneers. I would be remiss if I did not mention their names in this book. Dr. Selber of MDACC first developed latissimus dorsi flap reconstruction using a robotic surgical system. Dr. Toesca et al. at EIO of Milan first introduced robot-assisted nipple-sparing mastectomy and immediate prosthetic reconstruction. They motivated many breast surgeons. Following them, Dr. Sarfati of Gustave Roussy and I introduced different methods using robotic systems for the first time in France and Korea, respectively. Dr. Lai of CCH also developed an excellent training program for robotic breast surgery in Taiwan. These experts have made a great contributions to the development of robotic breast surgery.

I would like to thank Eun-Ji Kim, RN and Judy Ye-Jin Park, RN for their photo assistance in operating rooms and thank Elizabeth Burris and Ko Eun Park, MD for their advice for English manuscripts. I really appreciate the kind communication from Young Moon, RN, as well as the photos and information from the Severance Robot & MIS Center. I would like to express my gratitude to Intuitive Surgical Korea, Ethicon (Johnson & Johnson), Dalim Medical Corporation, Appliedmedical, RAPHA KOREA, Sejong Medical, and Medtronic for generously providing their product images for this book.

This book is written for breast surgeons or fellows who have not experienced surgery with robotic systems.

I hope this book will be a good friend to guide fellow surgeons all over the world into a new way of robotic breast surgery.

FEB 25, 2021

Hyung Seok Park MD, PhD

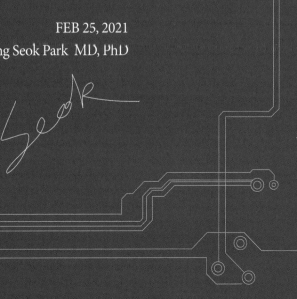

Jeea Lee MD

Clinical Research Assistant Professor
Department of Surgery, Yonsei University College of Medicine
Breast Cancer Center, Yonsei Cancer Center
Yonsei University Health System, Seoul, Korea

Haemin Lee MD

Clinical Research Assistant Professor
Department of Surgery, Yonsei University College of Medicine
Breast Cancer Center, Yonsei Cancer Center
Yonsei University Health System, Seoul, Korea

Dong Won Lee MD, PhD

Associate Professor
Department of Plastic and Reconstructive Surgery, Yonsei University College of Medicine
Breast Cancer Center, Yonsei Cancer Center
Yonsei University Health System, Seoul, Korea

Seung Yong Song MD, PhD

Associate Professor
Department of Plastic and Reconstructive Surgery, Yonsei University College of Medicine
Breast Cancer Center, Yonsei Cancer Center
Yonsei University Health System, Seoul, Korea

CONTENTS

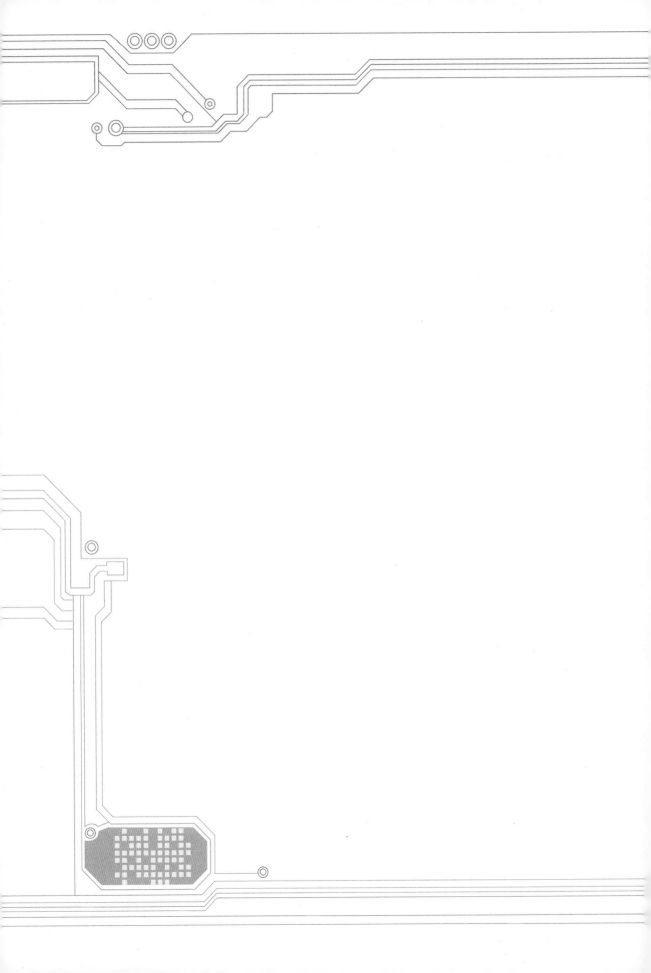

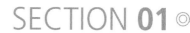

SECTION **01**

Introduction of Robotic Surgery

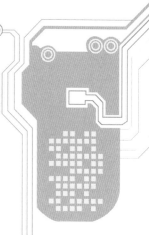

1. Robotic Surgical Systems

Hyung Seok Park and Haemin Lee

The robotic surgical system 'PUMA 560', a robotic surgical arm, was first used in a non-laparoscopic neurosurgical biopsy in 1985. The introduction of the robotic surgical system provided a great potential for endoscopic or laparoscopic surgery and aroused much interest among surgeons.[1]

The Automated Endoscopic System for Optimal Positioning (AESOP) system (Computer Motion, Goleta, California) was first approved by the FDA as a laparoscopic robotic surgical system. Using the AESOP system, the first robot laparoscopic cholecystectomy was introduced in 1987.[2] In Korea, the first attempt to use the AESOP 1000 system for cholecystectomy was reported at Severance Hospital in 1996.[2] However, the initial types of robotic surgical systems was widely used in Korea until the introduction of a new generation of robotic surgical systems because of the low cost-effectiveness and difficulty in use and training.[3]

In 2000, Intuitive Surgical Inc. introduced an innovative robotic surgical system encompassing surgical instruments and camera utensils named da Vinci. This system offers the precise "Endo-wrist" feature, which replicates the hands of skilled surgeons with greater degree of freedom compared to conventional laparoscopic or endoscopic devices in a small operative fields such as peritoneal cavity or non-visceral soft tissue spaces. The three dimensional magnification view in the camera provides a better view of the operative fields for surgeons to allow more delicate and meticulous tissue handling, suture, and dissection. The smaller robotic arm, compared to previous robotic systems, can minimize tissue injury, resulting in reduced surgical infections. These features improve surgical outcomes including hospital stay, post-operative pain, and quality of life.[4]

The generations of the da Vinci Surgical System

Intuitive Surgical Inc. has introduced four generations of the da Vinci Surgical System so far.

The da Vinci Standard is the first generation of the da Vinci®-Surgical System, introduced in 1999. It consists of three components: an ergonomically designed surgeon's console, a patient-side cart with four interactive robotic arms, and a high-performance vision system.

The second-generation da Vinci Surgical System was launched in 2006. The second generation system introduced a more enhanced 3D vision, updated user interface, and extended operating room integrations with advanced instruments. The enhanced 3D

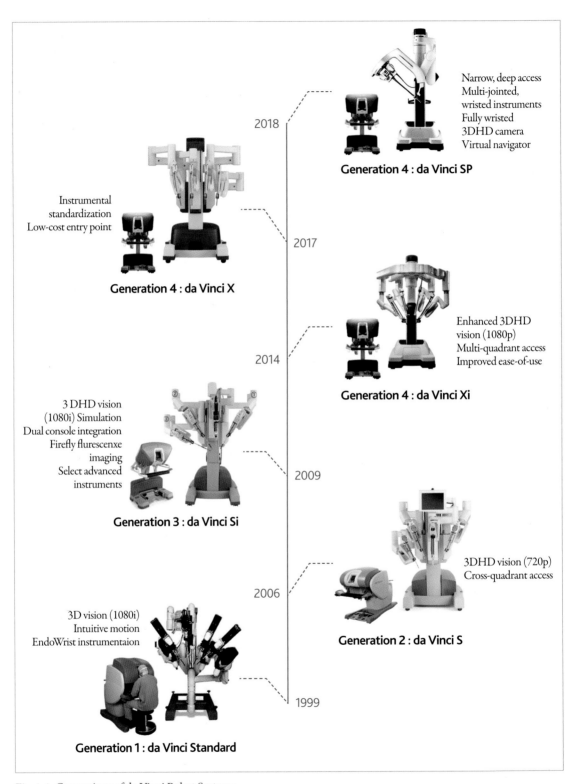

Fig. 1-1. Generations of da Vinci Robot Systems

vision provides up to 10 times magnification and an immersive view of the operative field.

The third-generation da Vinci Si was launched in 2009. It introduced dual-console capability. The Firefly fluorescence imaging technique became available.

The fourth-generation was introduced in 2014 with da Vinci Xi Surgical System. The da Vinci X was launched in 2017. The da Vinci X is a down-grade version of the Xi system, but it still has a much greater workspace than the Si system and enables focused-quadrant surgery. The da Vinci Xi has a rotating boom. The workspace is twice as wide as the X system. The boom in the Xi system provides multi-quadrant access, which is used for a variety of complex procedures.

The da Vinci SP Surgical System is the latest version of the fourth generation of the robot systems. It is designed for a single-port access with a single arm rotating 360 degrees with three multi-jointed instruments and a fully wristed 3DHD camera. Through a single 2.5 cm cannula, the da Vinci SP boom can rotate more than 360 degrees around the remote center of the cannula. The instrument cluster within the cannula also rotates over 360 degrees without any external collisions. It offers a reaching capability up to 24 cm deep in the operative field. It allows surgeons to triangulate instruments at the distal tip.[5,6]

REFERENCE

1. Kwoh YS, Hou J, Jonckheere EA, Hayati S. A robot with improved absolute positioning accuracy for CT guided stereotactic brain surgery. IEEE transactions on bio-medical engineering. 1988;35(2):153-60.

2. Lee W-J. Ten-year Experience of the da Vinci Robotic Surgery At Severance Yonsei University Hospital in Korea. Hanyang Med Rev. 2016;36(4):215-24.

3. Lee WJ, Hyung WJ, Rha K, Kim J, Song HJ, Lee YA, et al. Current experiences with robotic surgery at Severance Hospital, Yonsei University in Korea. Asian Journal of Endoscopic Surgery. 2010;3:8-13.

4. Leal Ghezzi T, Campos Corleta O. 30 Years of Robotic Surgery. World Journal of Surgery. 2016;40(10):2550-7.

5. Intuitive. da Vinci Surgery Coustomer Portal: Intuitive Surgical; 2019 [cited 2019. Available from: https://www.davincisurgerycommunity.com]

6. Intuitive. Intuitive, da Vinci, Robotic Surgical System: Intuitive Surgical; 2019 [cited 2019. Available from: https://www.intuitive.com/en-us/products-and-services/da-vinci.]

2. Development of Robotic Mastectomy

Hyung Seok Park

The first report of the robotic breast surgery was latissimus dorsi (LD) flap harvest for breast reconstruction in 2012 by Selber et al.[1] He performed three pedicled flaps for immediate implant-based breast reconstruction after nipple-sparing mastectomies and two reconstructions using pedicled flaps for radiated breasts during exchange of the expanders for implants through a minimal incision hidden in the axilla.[1] This report inspired a few surgeons to lead and develop a further application of robotic surgical systems in breast surgery.

My team at Severance Hospital began cadaveric labs for robotic mastectomy and immediate reconstruction using LD flap in 2013. Three experiences with the cadaveric labs provided a useful insight into robotic mastectomy and immediate reconstruction. However, the actual application of robotic mastectomy and immediate reconstruction as a clinical practice was not easy to perform due to the difficulty in patient enrollment. It is difficult to persuade patients to undergo the first attempt of a new procedure. Our

team failed to get consent for mastectomy and immediate reconstruction using robotic surgical system for three years.

In the meantime, Toesca et al. at European Institute of Oncology (EIO) in Milan first introduced robotic mastectomy and immediate reconstruction in 2017. They reported robotic mastectomy and immediate prosthetic reconstruction for the first time. In this report, they performed three contralateral risk-reducing nipple-sparing mastectomies and immediate breast reconstructions through a single port device inserted into the 2.5 cm axillary incision using da Vinci S (Intuitive Surgical Inc., Sunnyvale, CA). There were self-resolving neuropraxia and mild ecchymosis from electrocauterization; however, no long-term complications were observed.[2] After that, Sarfati et al. at Gustave Roussy in Paris reported a successful application of the da Vinci Xi system for risk-reducing nipple-sparing mastectomy and immediate reconstruction for a woman with *BRCA* mutation in 2018.[3] These reports encouraged my team to apply robotic surgical systems to mastectomy and immediate reconstruction in 2016 for the first time in Asia. My team developed a gasless technique with Chung's self-retractor, used in endoscopic/robotic trans-axillary thyroidectomy, for mastectomy using robotic surgical systems.[4] Following these reports of successful applications of robotic surgical systems, several other pioneers, including Lai et al. at Changhua Christian Hospital, Cheng et al. at Shin Kong

Wu Ho-su Memorial Hospital, Kuo et al. at LinKou Chang Gung Memorial Hospital in Taiwan, and Houvenaeghel et al. at Institut Paoli Calmettes in Marseille, reported their initial experience of robotic mastectomy.[5-8]

REFERENCES

1. Selber JC, Baumann DP, Holsinger FC. Robotic latissimus dorsi muscle harvest: a case series. Plastic and reconstructive surgery. 2012;129(6):1305-12.

2. Toesca A, Peradze N, Galimberti V, Manconi A, Intra M, Gentilini O, et al. Robotic Nipple-sparing Mastectomy and Immediate Breast Reconstruction With Implant: First Report of Surgical Technique. Annals of surgery. 2017;266(2):e28-e30.

3. Sarfati B, Honart JF, Leymarie N, Rimareix F, Al Khashnam H, Kolb F. Robotic da Vinci Xi-assisted nipple-sparing mastectomy: First clinical report. The breast journal. 2018;24(3):373-6.

4. Park HS, Kim JH, Lee DW, Song SY, Park S, Kim SI, et al. Gasless Robot-Assisted Nipple-Sparing Mastectomy: A Case Report. Journal of breast cancer. 2018;21(3):334-8.

5. Cheng F, editor Embracing minimally invasive surgery: the era of endoscopic and robotic breast surgery. International Endoscopic and Robotic Breast Surgery Symposium; 2019; Taiwan. Taiwan 2019.

6. Houvenaeghel G, Bannier M, Rua S, Barrou J, Heinemann M, Knight S, et al. Robotic breast and reconstructive surgery: 100 procedures in 2-years for 80 patients. Surgical oncology. 2019;31:38-45.

7. Kuo W-L, Huang J-J, Huang Y-T, Chueh L-F, Lee J-T, Tsai H-P, et al. Robot-assisted Mastectomy Followed by Immediate Autologous Microsurgical Free Flap Reconstruction: Techniques and Feasibility in Three Different Breast Cancer Surgical Scenarios. Clinical Breast Cancer. 2019.

8. Lai HW, Lin SL, Chen ST, Chen SL, Lin YL, Chen DR, et al. Robotic Nipple-sparing Mastectomy and Immediate Breast Reconstruction with Gel Implant. Plastic and reconstructive surgery Global open. 2018;6(6):e1828.

3. Current Evidences for Robotic Mastectomy

Hyung Seok Park and Jeea Lee

Since Toesca et al. presented the first robotic nipple-sparing mastectomy and immediate breast reconstruction with an implant, other studies of robotic mastectomy or breast reconstruction have been reported in the world.[1-8] Sarfati et al. conducted a prospective study with *BRCA* mutation carriers to evaluate the safety and feasibility of the robot system for prophylactic mastectomy.[7] Park et al. first introduced various methods of RNSM using gasless techniques or single port systems.[5] Lai et al. compared the surgical outcomes and learning curve between RNSM and endoscopic NSM (ENSM) in a case-control comparison study in 2020.[9] Cheng presented the initial experience of RNSM without prior ENSM experience.[1] Kuo et al. published three cases of free flap breast reconstruction for robot assisted mastectomy to show the wider clinical applications of robotic surgical systems to breast cancer.[3] Houvenaeghel et al. proposed the possible indications for RNSM including those who underwent RNSM with prosthetic or autologous reconstruction after neoadjuvant chemotherapy or previous radiotherapy. In 2019, Toesca et al. first reported the oncologic safety of robotic mastectomy with a short-term follow-up. In those studies, all authors agreed with the need for a long-term prospective study with a larger sample size.

In 2019, a panel of internationally representative experts participated in the generation of a consensus statement on robotic mastectomy. They discussed establishing standardized guidelines for robotic mastectomy and agreed on 52 consensus statements in 6 domains including indications, contraindications, technical considerations, patient counseling, outcome measures and indicators, and training and learning curve assessment.[9]

Table 3-1. Current Studies of Robotic Mastectomy and Immediate Reconstruction

Study (years)	Type of study	N	Age (years, range)	Indications (n [%])	Methods
Toesca (2019)[10]	Prospective	94	42 (24–59)	Ca ductal 30 (31.9%) Ca lobular 6 (6.4%) Infiltrating 3 (3.2%) In Situ 21 (22.3%) Prophylactic 34 (36.2%)	Gas
Sarfati (2018)[7]	Prospective	63	37 (24–52)	Prophylactic 62 (98.4%) Therapeutic 1 (1.6%)	Gas
Park (2019)[6]	Retrospective	12	46 (29–51)	Benign 2 (16.7%) DCIS 1 (8.3%) IDC 9 (75%)	Gas 2 (16.7%) Gasless 10 (83.3%)
Lai (2020)[9]	Prospective	131	48±8*	Therapeutic 131	RNSM 40 ENSM 91
Cheng (2019)[1]	Retrospective	47	N/A	N/A	Gas
Kou (2019)[3]	Retrospective	3	32–37	DCIS 2 IDC 1	RNSM 2 RSSM 1
Houvenaeghel (2019)[2]	Prospective	100	53.3 (21–83)	Primary Cancer 58 Local Recurrence 21 Prophylactic 1	RLDFR 73 (witn concomitant RM 26) RM 8

Study (years)	Reconstruction	Robotic surgical time (min)	Breast weight (g)	Complications
Toesca (2019)	DTI 84(89.4%) T/E 10(10.6%)	120 (47–230)	N/A	Infection 2 (2.1%), Hematoma 4 (4.3%), Necrosis 1 (1.1%), Axillary Web Syndrome 1 (1.1%), Implant Exposure 1 (1.1%), Eschar 4 (4.3%), Seroma 5 (5.3%), Erythema 1 (1.1%), Implant loss 2 (2.1%)
Sarfati (2018)	DTI 55 T/E 8	N/A	78–330	Open conversion 1 (1.6%), Infection 3 (4.8%), Neurapraxia 1 (1.6%), Implant rotation 1 (1.6%)
Park (2019)	DTI 3 (25%) T/E 9 (75%)	351 (267–480)	225.5 (150–436)	Skin Ischemia 2 (16.7%), Nipple Ischemia 1 (8.3%)
Lai (2020)	DTI (131, 100%)	241±61*	286±108*	Delayed Axillary Wound Healing 2 (5%), Partial Nipple Ischemia 1 (2.5%). Seroma 2 (5%), Blister 2 (5%), Skin Ischemia 2 (5%)
Cheng (2019)	N/A	N/A	N/A	N/A
Kou (2019)	PAP 2 DIEP 1	88 (73–125)	201 (130–272)	N/A
Houvenaeghel (2019)	RLDF 40 non–autologous LDF 5 RLDF+implant 28 Implant 7	301 (127–495)	330 (80–1500)	Hematoma 11, Infection 2, Blistering 10

*Mean Value, Ca, carcinoma; DCIS, ductal carcinoma in situ; DTI, direct–to–implant; IDC, invasive ductal carcinoma; RNSM, robotic nipple–sparing mastectomy; ENSM, endoscopic nipple–sparing mastectomy; RSSM, robotic skin–sparing mastectomy; RLDFR, Robotic latissimus dorsi flap reconstruction; RM, robotic mastectomy; T/E, tissue expander; PAP, profunda artery perforator; DIEP, deep inferior epigastric flaps.

REFERECES

1. Cheng F, editor Embracing minimally invasive surgery: the era of endoscopic and robotic breast surgery. International Endoscopic and Robotic Breast Surgery Symposium; 2019; Taiwan. Taiwan 2019.

2. Houvenaeghel G, Bannier M, Rua S, Barrou J, Heinemann M, Knight S, et al. Robotic breast and reconstructive surgery: 100 procedures in 2-years for 80 patients. Surgical oncology. 2019;31:38-45.

3. Kuo W-L, Huang J-J, Huang Y-T, Chueh L-F, Lee J-T, Tsai H-P, et al. Robot-assisted Mastectomy Followed by Immediate Autologous Microsurgical Free Flap Reconstruction: Techniques and Feasibility in Three Different Breast Cancer Surgical Scenarios. Clinical Breast Cancer. 2019.

4. Lai HW, Toesca A, Sarfati B, Park HS, Houvenaeghel G, Selber JC, et al. Consensus Statement on Robotic Mastectomy-Expert Panel From International Endoscopic and Robotic Breast Surgery Symposium (IERBS) 2019. Annals of surgery. 2020.

5. Park HS, Kim JH, Lee DW, Song SY, Park S, Kim SI, et al. Gasless Robot-Assisted Nipple-Sparing Mastectomy: A Case Report. Journal of breast cancer. 2018;21(3):334-8.

6. Park HS, Lee J, Lee DW, Song SY, Lew DH, Kim SI, et al. Robot-assisted Nipple-sparing Mastectomy with Immediate Breast Reconstruction: An Initial Experience. Scientific reports. 2019;9(1):15669.

7. Sarfati B, Struk S, Leymarie N, Honart JF, Alkhashnam H, Tran de Fremicourt K, et al. Robotic Prophylactic Nipple-Sparing Mastectomy with Immediate Prosthetic Breast Reconstruction: A Prospective Study. Annals of surgical oncology. 2018;25(9):2579-86.

8. Toesca A, Peradze N, Galimberti V, Manconi A, Intra M, Gentilini O, et al. Robotic Nipple-sparing Mastectomy and Immediate Breast Reconstruction With Implant: First Report of Surgical Technique. Annals of surgery. 2017;266(2):e28-e30.

9. Lai H-W, Chen S-T, Tai C-M, Lin S-L, Lin Y-J, Huang R-H, et al. Robotic- Versus Endoscopic-Assisted Nipple-Sparing Mastectomy with Immediate Prosthesis Breast Reconstruction in the Management of Breast Cancer: A Case–Control Comparison Study with Analysis of Clinical Outcomes, Learning Curve, Patient-Reported Aesthetic Results, and Medical Cost. Annals of surgical oncology. 2020.

10. Toesca A, Invento A, Massari G, Girardi A, Peradze N, Lissidini G, Sangalli C, Maisonneuve P, Manconi A, Gottardi A, Baker JL, Bottiglieri L, Naninato P, Farante G, Magnoni F, De Scalzi A, Corso G, Colleoni M, De Lorenzi F, Sacchini V, Galimberti V, Intra M, Rietjens M, Veronesi P. Update on the Feasibility and Progress on Robotic Breast Surgery. Ann Surg Oncol. 2019 Oct;26(10):3046-3051. doi: 10.1245/s10434-019-07590-7. Epub 2019 Jul 24. PMID: 31342391; PMCID: PMC7493284.

4. FDA Warning about Robotic Mastectomy

Hyung Seok Park

In Feb 2019, the FDA in the USA announced a safety communication urging caution when using robot-assisted surgical devices in women's health, including mastectomy and other cancer related surgeries with an exception of certain types of robotic surgery.[1] The communication includes ten headings: audience, medical specialties, device, purpose, summary of problem and scope, recommendations for patients, recommendations for health care providers, FDA actions, reporting problems to the FDA, other resources, and contact information. In brief, they insisted that the relative benefits and risks of surgeries using robotic surgical systems compared to conventional surgical method in cancer treatment and prevention have not been established. Particularly, they cited a study comparing a minimally-invasive surgery to an open conventional surgery in cervical cancer.[2] The study showed minimally-invasive surgery to be associated with a lower rate of long-term survival compared to open abdominal surgery. To date, the FDA has not cleared marketing authorization

for any robotic surgical systems for use of cancer treatment and prevention, including mastectomy, in the USA. This became a huge hurdle for the application of robotic surgical system in breast surgery for cancer treatment and prevention in the USA.

Even though the FDA insisted that there is a lack of evidence of safety and benefits of surgeries using robotic surgical systems, there are many reports of laparoscopic or endoscopic surgeries using robotic surgical systems for cancer patients.[1] Robotic surgical systems are being widely used for not only urologic cancer surgery but also other cancer related surgery including colorectal surgery, gastrectomy, hepatectomy, thyroidectomy, and even pancreaticoduodenectomy in many developed countries.[3-5] Pai et al. summarized the current evidence for the adoption of robotic total mesorectal excision for rectal cancer from various relevant studies.[5] Marano et al. conducted a systematic review with meta-analysis to determine the benefit of robotic surgery, and it demonstrated that robotic gastrectomy for gastric cancer reduces blood loss and hospital stays compared to laparoscopic and open gastrectomy.[4] Abood and Tsung analyzed robot-assisted liver resection, and it reported the feasibility and safety of minor and major robot-assisted liver resections in terms of estimated blood loss, length of stay, and complications.[3] Kim et al. demonstrated that robotic thyroidectomy provides higher satisfaction levels of the overall and cosmetic results to patients.[6] Guerrini et

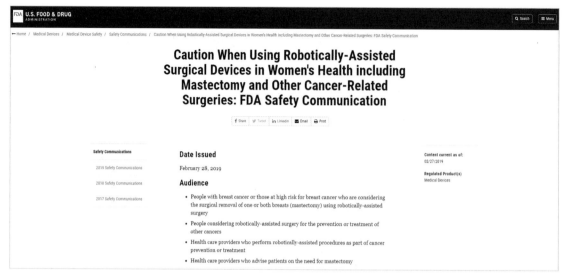

Fig. 4-1. The US FDA Caution on website (https://www.fda.gov/medical-devices/safety-communications/caution-when-using-robotically-assisted-surgical-devices-womens-health-including-mastectomy-and)

al. conducted a systematic review and meta-analysis of robotic and laprasopic distal pancreatectomy to show that the rate of spleen preservation increased, the risk of conversion to open surgery reduced, and the length of hospital stay was shorter in the robotic distal pancreatectomy group compared to the laparoscopic distal pancreatectomy group.[7] Many of these studies even reported cases of cancer surgery using robotic surgical system conducted in the U.S.A.[3, 5, 8, 9]

The principle of conventional nipple-sparing mastectomy (CNSM) is the preservation of the nipple-areolar complex (NAC) and skin of the breast and complete removal of breast parenchyma with proper margins of NAC. Robotic Nipple-Sparing mastectomy (RNSM) shares the same principle with that of the CNSM. Robot mastectomy basically secures safety margins by dissecting the superficial

and deep layer of the superficial fascia with a 3D magnified view and the precise movement of robotic arms. In addition, expert panels at the International Endoscopic and Robotic Breast Surgery Symposium (IERBS) 2019 in Taiwan strongly agreed that the indications of RNSM are not different from those of CNSM.[10]

Furthermore, Toesca et al. reported the short term oncologic safety and favorable 90-day post-operative complication rates in women who underwent RNSM.[11] A randomized clinical trial revealed no difference in complication rates as well as the high satisfaction and quality of life compared to CNSM, which represents definite advantages of RNSM.[12]

However, because there is still a lack of long-term outcomes and large sample sized prospective studies, caution should be made in the use of robotic surgical systems for mastectomy. For better application of RNSM, proper educational programs are necessary. The lack of well-designed educational programs for robotic surgery for trainees is one of the limitations of the wider application of RNSM. Severance Robot and MIS Center provides a basic try and animal skill labs for trainees who are preparing for robot breast surgery. The center can provide cadaveric skill labs for surgeons upon request to fulfill unmet needs. The next chapter will briefly introduce the educational programs offered by Severance Robot and MIS Center.

REFERENCE

1. U. S. Food & Drug administration F. Caution When Using Robotically-Assisted Surgical Devices in Women's Health including Mastectomy and Other Cancer-Related Surgeries: FDA Safety Communication. In: Education tDoIaC, editor. Silver Spring, MD2019.

2. Ramirez PT, Frumovitz M, Pareja R, Lopez A, Vieira M, Ribeiro R, et al. Minimally Invasive versus Abdominal Radical Hysterectomy for Cervical Cancer. New England Journal of Medicine. 2018;379(20):1895-904.

3. Abood GJ, Tsung A. Robot-assisted surgery: improved tool for major liver resections? Journal of hepato-biliary-pancreatic sciences. 2013;20(2):151-6.

4. Marano A, Choi YY, Hyung WJ, Kim YM, Kim J, Noh SH. Robotic versus Laparoscopic versus Open Gastrectomy: A Meta-Analysis. Journal of gastric cancer. 2013;13(3):136-48.

5. Pai A, Melich G, Marecik SJ, Park JJ, Prasad LM. Current status of robotic surgery for rectal cancer: A bird's eye view. Journal of minimal access surgery. 2015;11(1):29-34.

6. Kim WW, Jung JH, Lee J, Kang JG, Baek J, Lee WK, et al. Comparison of the Quality of Life for Thyroid Cancer Survivors Who Had Open Versus Robotic Thyroidectomy. Journal of laparoendoscopic & advanced surgical techniques Part A. 2016;26(8):618-24.

7. Guerrini GP, Lauretta A, Belluco C, Olivieri M, Forlin M, Basso S, et al. Robotic versus laparoscopic distal pancreatectomy: an up-to-date meta-analysis. BMC Surgery. 2017;17(1):105.

8. Mohamed SE, Saeed A, Moulthrop T, Kandil E. Retroauricular robotic thyroidectomy with concomitant neck-lift surgery. Annals of surgical oncology. 2015;22(1):172.

9. Sebastian R, Howell MH, Chang KH, Adrales G, Magnuson T, Schweitzer M, et al. Robot-assisted versus laparoscopic Roux-en-Y gastric bypass and sleeve gastrectomy: a propensity score-matched comparative analysis using the 2015-2016 MBSAQIP database. Surg Endosc. 2019;33(5):1600-12.

10. Lai HW, Toesca A, Sarfati B, Park HS, Houvenaeghel G, Selber JC, et al. Consensus Statement on Robotic Mastectomy-Expert Panel From International Endoscopic and Robotic Breast Surgery Symposium (IERBS) 2019. Annals of surgery. 2020.

11. Toesca A, Invento A, Massari G, Girardi A, Peradze N, Lissidini G, et al. Update on the Feasibility and Progress on Robotic Breast Surgery. Annals of surgical oncology. 2019;26(10):3046-51.

12. Toesca A, editor Recent progress in endoscopic breast surgery and robot-assisted mastectomy. Global Breast Cancer Conference 2019; 2019; Songdo ConvensiA, Incheon, Korea: Korean Breast Cancer Society; 2019.

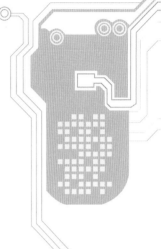

SECTION **02**

Preclinical Skill Lab and Perioperative Preparation

5. Preclinical Skill Lab for Robotic Mastectomy

Hyung Seok Park and Severance Robot and MIS Center

Introduction of Severance Robot and MIS Center

Systematic education and various experiences are essential elements to grow into a qualified surgeon. Standardized training programs have gained to promote safe and acceptable surgical outcomes, for sophisticated instruments and products, including robotic surgical systems have been applied to surgery more than before. Severance Hospital and Intuitive Surgical Inc. opened the Severance Robot and MIS (minimally-invasive surgery) Center (Fig 5-1) in 2008 to provide standardized education programs and develop well-trained surgeons and new surgical techniques in a diverse range of surgical specialties, including general surgery, urology, gynecology, cardio-thoracic surgery, otolaryngology, and neurosurgery.

This Severance Robot and MIS Center is the second training center in Asia to be validated by Intuitive Surgical Corporations. Many surgeons from various countries have visited and received specialized trainings and hands-on experiences of with surgical case observations and discussions with experienced surgeons. Its training capabilities enable surgeons, nurses, and operating room personnel to receive more systematic training, knowledge, and consulting services, including animal and cadaveric laboratories. This center has various training programs, such as simulator training, system training, case observation, and advanced courses. Here are some details about those programs. You can contact through the website or email for more information.

Case Observation

This course is designed to observe and discuss live surgery in the operating theater with the operator. Over 100 trainees come to take this course to develop clinical and technical skills annually. The strength of Severance Hospital is its diverse clinical departments, each of which is actively using and developing robotic surgical techniques.

Basic Training

The objective of this program is for surgeons and their patient-side assistants to learn and practice the robotic skills required to use robotic surgical systems safely and effectively. Throughout this program, surgeons learn and practice the operation of surgical robots using experimental animals as if performing on actual patients. This workshop is conducted in collaboration with robot manufacturing companies.

Advanced Course

This is a robotic surgery training program that was first designed by Severance Hospital. This is an advanced course for surgeons who have completed the Basic Training. This course develops specific robotic surgery skills for procedures like lower anterior resection, transoral robotic surgery, mastectomy, and the like. This course provides an opportunity to learn practical skills via case observations and skill practices using cadavers, which can be of a direct help in clinical settings.

Surgical Workshop

Severance Robot and MIS Center is well equipped with the optimal space and necessary equipment for skill labs so that surgeons can focus on developing their experiences and technical skills in laparoscopic surgery as well as robotic surgery.

Nurse Training

In this course, nurses learn how to operate and manage robotic surgical systems. Nurses have opportunities to observe in the operation theater to experience how the system is actually applied in clinical settings. Via this training, nurses can enhance their understanding of surgical robots and capabilities to set up an optimal environment for robotic surgery.

Others

1) Simulator training: This program is based on understanding the basic concepts of robotic systems and practicing the manipulation of the surgeon console and other instruments to get accustomed to the system.

2) Laparoscopic Training: By using a laparoscopic training box, trainees can learn how to deal with laparoscopic instruments and develop suture skills.

3) Visitor Program: This program is designed for students, residents, colleagues, and professors who are interested in robotic surgery. This program provides an opportunity to observe robotic surgery and experience surgical robots in the training center.

4) Severance Surgical Robot class: This is part of a social program organized by the Severance Robot and MIS Center, which has been regularly held since 2010. It is designed for children and young students to elevate their interests and understanding. The purpose of this program is to foster future talent in the surgical robot development industry by providing experiences of the surgical robot.

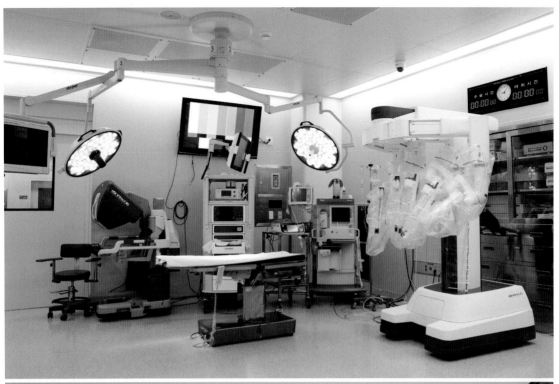

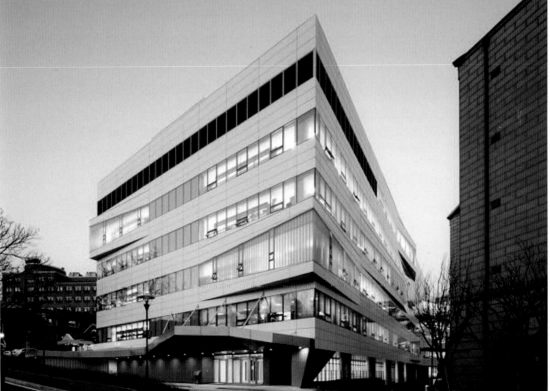

Fig. 5-1. Severance Robot and MIS Center

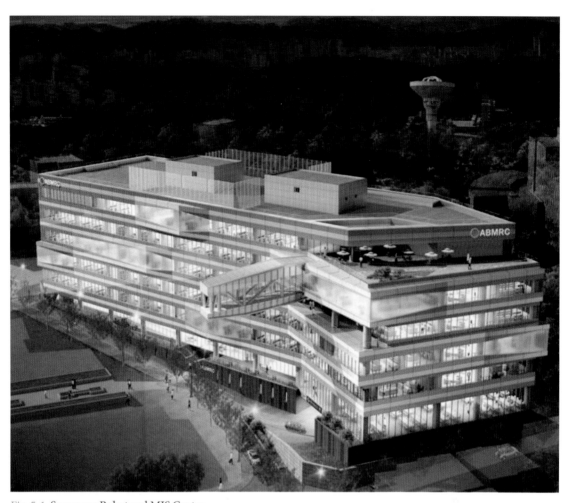

Fig. 5-1. Severance Robot and MIS Center

50-1 Yonsei-ro, Seodaemun-gu, Seoul 03722, Korea
- Tel: 82-2-2228-6320
- Fax: 82-2-312-2538
- E-mail: robotcenter@yuhs.ac
- Website: http://robotmis.iseverance.com

6. Candidate Selection for Robotic Mastectomy

Hyung Seok Park

The selection of the candidates for RNSM is similar to that for CNSM. Tumor involvement of the nipple-areolar complex or skin is a contraindication for RNSM. If there is an equivocal lesion of tumor involvement into the nipple-areolar complex or skin in preoperative imaging studies, an intraoperative frozen biopsy can help to identify the tumor involvement. If tumor involvement is identified by the frozen biopsy, I recommend an additional resection of the superficial margin, NAC, or skin to achieve safety margins. If the permanent pathology reveals tumor involvement of the margins, additional dissection should be performed in a 2nd-stage operation. Adjuvant radiation may be an alternative option for superficial margin or NAC focal involvement. A multidisciplinary team approach and shared decision-making with patients should be taken for this issue.

To select good candidates for RNSM, high risk factors of nipple or skin necrosis should be considered before surgery. Prior operative scars in the overlying breast skin or NAC can deteriorate blood supply of the dermal layer,

and it thus can increase the risk of nipple and skin necrosis.[1] Age[2], BMI[3] or co-morbidities such as smoking habit[4], hypertension[5], diabetes mellitus[6], types of incision, thickness of the skin flap[7], the volume of the breast[2] are also risk factors of nipple and skin necrosis. History of previous radiation should be checked, for radiation therapy may induce fibrosis or capsular contracture[8] of implant-based reconstruction.

Herein, the consensus statement developed as the standardized guidelines on robotic mastectomy by representative expert panel of 10 surgeons during the International Endoscopic and Robotic Breast Surgery Symposium (IERBS) 2019 suggests the indications and contraindications as shown in the following table. Women with small to moderate breast size below cup size C and tumor size of T3 and below are suitable for robotic mastectomy. The statement recommends that women with adequate tumor-skin distance of at least 3 mm with no nipple-areolar complex involvement on preoperative imaging, and no clinical and radiological evidence of skin involvement are appropriate candidates for robotic mastectomy.[9]

REFERENCES

1. Jensen JA, Orringer JS, Giuliano AE. Nipple-Sparing Mastectomy in 99 Patients With a Mean Follow-up of 5 Years. Annals of Surgical Oncology. 2011;18(6):1665-70.

2. Chirappapha P, Petit JY, Rietjens M, De Lorenzi F, Garusi C, Martella S, et al. Nipple-Sparing mastectomy: does breast morphological factor related to necrotic complications? Plastic and reconstructive surgery Global open. 2014;2(1):e99.

Table 6-1. Final Consensus Final Consensus Statements on Robotic Mastectomy With Modified Delphi Methodology (Indications and contraindications)

Domains	Sub–domains	Statements
Indications	Patient factors	1. Robotic mastecomy is suitable for women with small to moderate breast size 2. Robotic mastecomy is suitable for women with breast cup size C and below
	Disease factors	3. Robotic mastecomy is suitable for women with clinical tumor size of up 5 cm (T3 and below), with adequate tumor–skin distance of at least 3 mm and above with no NAC involvment in preperative imaging 4. Robotic mastecomy is suitable for women with breast cancer up to clinical stage ⅢA (up to T3, N1–2) with cautious considerations in selected cases with adequate response to neoadjuvant therapy and possible suboptimal cosmesis informed to patient in view of need for adjuvant radiotherapy 5. Robotic mastecomy is suitable for women requiring sentinel lymph node biopsy, where radioisotope alone is sufficient except in selected cases with neoadjuvant chemotherapy, dual modality is advised 6. Robotic mastecomy is suitable for women with clinically node negative disease 7. Robotic mastecomy is suitable for women with low disease burden in the axilla in selected cases with good tumor biology such as luminal A subtype or micro–metastasis on sentinel lymph node biopsy 8. Robotic mastecomy is suitable for women with no clinical and radiological evidence of skin involvement 9. Robotic mastecomy is suitable for women with tumor in any quadrants
	Prophylactic	10. Robotic mastecomy is suitable for women indicated for prophylactic mastectomy
Contraindications	Patient factors	11. Robotic mastecomy is not contraindicated but less than ideal and technically challenging for women with ptotic breast or cup size D and above in view of possible suboptmal cosmesis in cases of either direct–to–implant reconstruction or absence of contra–lateral mastopexy/reduction mammolasty 12. Robotic mastecomy is not recommended during the initial learning curve for women with poor performance status and multiple co–morbidities in view of possibe long operation time to avoid risks of post–op complications
	Disease factors	13. Robotic mastecomy is not recommended for women with clinical NAC involvement, as the main indication for robotic mastecomy is total skin and Nipple–Sparing mastectomy 14. Robotic mastecomy is not recommended for women with inflammatory breast cancer or T4d lesion 15. Robotic mastecomy is not recommended for women with clinical of skin involvement or T4d lesion 16. Direct–to–implant reconstruction is possible but ideal for women with clinical or radiological evidence of pectoralis major involvement, with the premise reconstruction 17. Robotic mastecomy is not recommended for women with clinical or radiological evidence of chest wall invasion
	Out of indications	18. Robotic mastecomy is not recommended for indications other than stated in this consensus statements until at least a Level III and above evidence is available.

Adapted from Lai et al. Ann. Surg. June 2020–Volume 271–Issue 6–p1005–1012, with permission of Wolters Kluwer Health, Inc.[9]

3. Davies K, Allan L, Roblin P, Ross D, Farhadi J. Factors affecting post-operative complications following skin sparing mastectomy with immediate breast reconstruction. Breast (Edinburgh, Scotland). 2011;20(1):21-5.

4. Algaithy ZK, Petit JY, Lohsiriwat V, Maisonneuve P, Rey PC, Baros N, et al. Nipple-Sparing mastectomy: can we predict the factors predisposing to necrosis? European journal of surgical oncology: the journal of the European Society of Surgical Oncology and the British Association of Surgical Oncology. 2012;38(2):125-9.

5. McCarthy CM, Mehrara BJ, Riedel E, Davidge K, Hinson A, Disa JJ, et al. Predicting complications following expander/implant breast reconstruction: an outcomes analysis based on preoperative clinical risk. Plastic and reconstructive surgery. 2008;121(6):1886-92.

6. Hultman CS, Daiza S. Skin-sparing mastectomy flap com-

plications after breast reconstruction: review of incidence, management, and outcome. Annals of plastic surgery. 2003;50(3):249-55; discussion 55.

7. Garwood ER, Moore D, Ewing C, Hwang ES, Alvarado M, Foster RD, et al. Total skin-sparing mastectomy: complications and local recurrence rates in 2 cohorts of patients. Annals of surgery. 2009;249(1):26-32.

8. Rosato RM, Dowden RV. Radiation therapy as a cause of capsular contracture. Annals of plastic surgery. 1994; 32(4):342-5.

9. Lai HW, Toesca A, Sarfati B, Park HS, Houvenaeghel G, Selber JC, et al. Consensus Statement on Robotic Mastectomy-Expert Panel From International Endoscopic and Robotic Breast Surgery Symposium (IERBS) 2019. Annals of surgery. 2020.

7. Preparation at Ward for Robotic Mastectomy

Hyung Seok Park

Informed Consent

General considerations of the nipple-sparing mastectomy and immediate reconstruction including headings (purpose, outcomes, process, methods, estimated time, possible complications of RNSM, other treatment options, etc.) should be included in the written informed consent. Also, the written informed consent at my institution provides an information of the FDA recommendation for health care providers. There are seven recommendations for health care providers in the FDA safety communication.

In brief, it recommends that patients understand that the FDA has not cleared and approved robotic surgical systems in use of cancer-related surgeries in the USA due to the lack of oncologic outcomes. However, you can explain that there are some early reports on short-term oncologic safety and post-operative complication rates from studies in other countries.

The FDA has approved robotic surgical systems in certain types of surgery, like robotic prostatectomy, for example, but not yet for mastectomy. The FDA recommends appropriate training for the use of robotic surgical systems. Specific training experience in skill labs and fellowship training for breast and robotic surgery are offered by several educational programs, such as observational and educational programs at Severance Robot and MIS Center. It is best to inform patients about your experience, training, and expected outcomes in robotic surgery and mastectomy. For the purpose of a shared decision-making, information concerning the benefits, risks, and all available alternative treatment options should be provided to patients. The FDA has oversight of clinical studies conducted in the USA that involve legally marketed robotic surgical systems to investigate a new intended utility. For the use of robotic surgical systems for mastectomy in the USA, report to the FDA's investigational device exemption (IDE) website (https://www.fda.gov/medical-devices/how-study-and-market-your-device/device-advice-investigational-device-exemption-ide).

You can provide information about adverse effects or complications of robotic surgical systems to the website provided by the FDA (https://www.fda.gov/safety/reporting-serious-problems-fda/reporting-health-professionals).

For health care providers outside of the USA, please check your domestic regulations for robotic surgical systems in the use of mastectomy.

수술[시술, 검사], 수혈 동의서

(선택진료 신청 포함)

수술(시술/검사) 설명

1. 수술(시술/검사)의 목적 및 효과

로봇을 이용한 유방암 수술로서 본 수술의 목적은 유방암을 제거하고, 액와 림프절 전이 여부 확인 및 병기(병의 진행 정도)를 평가하여 향후 보조 치료 시행 여부 및 방법(방사선 치료, 항암 약물 치료, 항암 호르몬 치료, 표적 치료)을 결정하고 예후를 예측하기 위함입니다. 로봇수술은 최소침습 수술법으로 수술 기법이 재발의 확률을 줄일 수 있는 것은 아닙니다. 로봇수술의 유익성은 겨드랑이에 3-6cm 정도의 절개창을 통해 수술을 진행하여 기존 수술방법과 달리 수술 흉터가 눈에 띄지 않는 곳에 위치하게 됩니다. 10배 이상의 확대된 3차원 영상을 통해 미세한 해부학적 구조를 더욱 정확히 식별할 수 있고 로봇 팔을 이용해 정교한 움직임을 가능하게 하여 수술을 보다 용이하게 할 수 있습니다.

2. 수술(시술/검사) 과정 및 방법, 부위 및 추정 소요시간

1) 유방 전 절제술

유방전체 조직을 제거하는 수술로 보존하는 구조에 따라 다음과 같은 종류로 나눌 수 있습니다.

가. 유두보존 유방 전 절제술

유두와 피부를 모두 남기고 유방 조직만을 모두 제거하는 방법입니다. 유두 밑에 유방조직이 어느 정도 남기 때문에 유방암의 재발가능성이 약간 올라간다는 단점이 있지만, 자신의 유두와 피부가 모두 남기 때문에 유방 재건수술 후 인공 유두에 비해 자연스럽다는 장점이 있어, 최근 들어 유방암 수술에 많이 이용되고 있습니다.

나. 피부보존 유방 전 절제술

유방 조직을 덮고 있는 피부를 제외하고 유방 조직 및 유두를 제거하는 수술입니다. 제거된 유두는 인공적으로 성형할 수 있습니다.

다. 근치 유방 전 절제술

유방 및 유방 조직을 덮고 있는 피부와 유두부위를 모두 제거하는 방법으로 로봇을 이용하지 않고 기존의 고식적인 개방적 방법을 이용한 수술입니다. 로봇수술 중 피부나 유두-유륜 복합체나 피부를 보존하지 못한다고 판단되면 로봇을 사용하지 않고 근치 유방 전절제술로 전환될 수 있습니다.

2) 액와부 수술

가. 감시 림프절 생검

감시 림프절이란 유방암이 액와 림프절로 전이할 때 처음으로 도달하는 림프절로서, 수술 중 이 림프절에 유방암의 전이가 확인될 경우 추가적으로 액와 림프절 곽청술을 시행하게 됩니다. 수술 전에 방사성 동위원소나 생체 염료를 유방에 주사하여 감시 림프절을 표시하고 수술 중에 생검합니다.

나. 액와 림프절 곽청술

액와 림프절 곽청술은 액와부 피부 아래 림프절부터 소흉근 하단부(레벨 II) 림프절까지 제거하는 수술이며, 감시 림프절에서 전이가 확인되었거나, 수술 전 검사에서 림프절의 전이가 확인되었을 경우 시행하게 됩니다.

Fig. 7-1. An example of the informed consent (Korean)

3) 수술 과정

　　가. 전신마취 하에 겨드랑이에 3-6cm 정도 피부를 절개합니다. 환자에 따라 절개창의
　　　　길이는 변할 수 있습니다.

　　나. 액와부 수술은 동위원소나 생체 염료를 함유한 림프절을 찾아 실시하며 동결절편
　　　　조직검사를 통해 전이여부를 확인합니다. 만약 전이가 확인되면 액와 림프절 곽청
　　　　술을 추가적으로 시행하게 되며, 전이가 되지 않은 경우 액와 림프절 곽청술은 시
　　　　행하지 않습니다.

　　다. 로봇을 이용하여 겨드랑이 절개창을 통해 유방조직을 피하 조직과 흉벽에서 박리
　　　　하여 제거합니다.

　　라. 수술부위를 지혈하고 유방절제술이 종료되면, 재건수술이 계획된 경우 재건수술을
　　　　시도 합니다.

4) 수술 시간

마취 및 수술 준비 시간을 제외하고 수술에 소요되는 시간은 약 2-4시간 정도이며 수술 중 동결
절편검사 시행여부와 환자 상태, 수술방법의 변경, 수술장 소견에 따라 차이가 있을 수 있습니다.

3. 발현 가능한 합병증의 내용, 정도 및 대처 방법

　1) **전신 마취에 따른 합병증**

　　: 폐렴, 무기폐, 기흉, 마취제 과민반응 등

　2) **수술부위의 출혈**

　　: 일반적으로 모든 수술은 수술 후 출혈의 가능성을 가지고 있습니다. 특히 수술 전
　　항혈소판제제 (아스피린 등)나 항응고제제 등을 복용한 경우에는 출혈 위험성이
　　증가하므로 수술 전에 이러한 약제들의 복용에 관하여 담당 주치의와 상담을 통해서
　　조절을 받아야 합니다. 미세한 출혈의 경우에는 수술부위의 압박으로 지혈하며 출혈량에
　　따라서 재수술이나 수혈을 요할 수도 있습니다.

　3) **상처부위 감염, 장액종, 괴사 형성**

　　: 수술 후 상처 부위 감염, 장액종, 괴사 형성이 될 수 있습니다. 창상감염이 되는 경우
　　항생제 치료가 필요할 수 있고, 수술 후 장액종이 고인 경우 수 차례 주사기로 흡인할
　　수 있습니다. 수술 후 상처부위 피부 허혈 및 괴사가 발생할 수 있습니다. 상처 부위
　　합병증의 경우 고령, 흡연 과거력, 유방의 부피가 커서 절제범위가 넓은 경우 발생
　　위험이 높다고 알려져 있습니다. 수술 중 사용하는 전기소작기 혹은 혈관봉합기에서
　　발생하는 열에 의해 피부에 온열손상 혹은 피부괴사가 발생할 수 있습니다. 대부분
　　보존적 치료로 해결될 수 있으며, 상처 부위 합병증으로 인해 상처 회복이 더디거나,
　　상피화로 회복이 안 될 경우 손상피부 절제 후 추가 봉합이 필요할 수 있습니다. 이
　　경우 추가 봉합 부위의 추가적인 흉터가 발생할 수 있습니다.

　4) **유두-유륜 복합체 괴사 가능성**

　　: 유두-유륜 복합체를 보존할 경우 혈액 순환 장애로 괴사가 있을 수 있습니다.
　　부분괴사가 발생한 경우 특별한 치료 없이 회복되는 경우도 있으나 괴사정도에 따라
　　심한 경우 유두-유륜 복합체를 절제하고 인공유두를 만드는 수술이 필요할 수
　　있습니다.

　5) **액와부 림프절 절제 시 작은 신경 가지의 절제 가능성**

Fig. 7-1. An example of the informed consent (Korean)

INFORMED CONSENT FOR
ROBOTIC BREAST CANCER SURGERY

1. Purpose and Outcome of Operation

There are three main purpose of breast cancer surgery including conventional and robotic surgery. The first is to remove breast cancer. The second is to determine whether to perform adjuvant therapy and which therapeutic methods should be used (e.g., radiation therapy, chemotherapy, hormone therapy, or targeted therapy). The third is to predict the prognosis by evaluating the stage (progress of disease) including tumor size and lymph node metastasis. Robotic surgery is a form of minimally invasive surgery and as a technique, it does not reduce the probability of recurrence. The benefit of robotic surgery is that, unlike existing surgical procedures, the surgical scar is placed in an inconspicuous place because the operation is performed through an incision measuring 3-6 cm in an armpit. Tiny anatomical structures can be identified more accurately through the x10 magnification of three-dimensional images, and the surgical procedure itself is facilitated by the robot arms, which enable delicate movements.

2. Operation Process, Method, Region, and Estimated Time

1) Total Mastectomy

Mastectomy, which is surgery performed to eliminate the entirety of breast tissue, can be classified as follows according to the structures that are preserved.

A. Nipple-sparing Mastectomy

This is a method to eliminate all breast tissue, leaving the nipple and skin. As a small amount of breast tissue remains below the nipple, the risk of recurrence of breast cancer increases slightly. However, because both the nipple and skin remain present after surgery, the breast has a more natural appearance than when an artificial nipple is used. Therefore, this technique is widely used in breast cancer surgery.

B. Skin-sparing Mastectomy

This procedure eliminates the breast tissue and nipple, except for the skin covering the breast. The removed nipple can be recreated artificially.

C. (Modified) Radical Mastectomy

This is not robotic surgery; instead, it uses an existing conventional open method to eliminate all skin covering the breast, the nipple area, and all breast tissue. If it is judged that the skin or nipple-areolar complex (NAC) can not be preserved during robotic surgery, the surgery can be converted to modified radical mastectomy, with no further use of the robot.

2) Axillary Surgery

A. Sentinel Lymph Node Biopsy

The sentinel node is the lymph node where breast cancer first arrives when it spreads to the axillary lymph nodes. Radioactive isotopes or biological dyes are injected into the breast before surgery to mark sentinel nodes and a biopsy is performed during surgery. When the spread of breast cancer to a sentinel lymph node is confirmed during surgery, axillary lymph node dissection is additionally performed.

B. Axillary Lymph Node Dissection

Axillary lymph node dissection is a surgical procedure to remove lymph nodes, extending from below the axillary skin to the lower part of the pectoralis minor (level II). It is performed when metastasis is confirmed in a sentinel node or when lymph node metastasis is confirmed through an examination before surgery.

3) Surgical Procedure

A. 3- to 6-cm incision in the armpit skin is made under general anesthesia. The length of the incision varies

Fig. 7-2. An example of the informed consent (English)

movement due to severe pain after surgery. Rehabilitation treatment can be conducted jointly with the Department of Rehabilitation Medicine.

7) Lymphedema of the Upper Limbs Such As the Arms and Hands
Lymphedema of the upper limbs and severe resultant pain can occur due to axillary lymph node dissection. To prevent this, a massage can be performed. If lymphedema occurs, the use of compression stockings or rehabilitation treatment can be considered if needed.

8) Complications Caused by Injection of Carbon Dioxide Gas
When carbon dioxide gas is injected to secure a space for the surgical operation during robotic surgery, subcutaneous emphysema can occur. When injecting the gas, hypercapnia can also occur due to absorption of the gas into blood vessels. In such cases, the gas injection should be stopped and conservative treatment can be tried by adjusting the ventilation through the respirator. In severe cases, this complication can induce a carbon dioxide embolism. In such a case, the gas injection should be stopped immediately and conservative techniques that induce blood vessel gas emission are performed, or the surgical method is changed.

9) Risk due to the Surgical Robot
No established risk related to the surgical robot has been reported. However, physical damage can occur due to errors during its use.
Furthermore, accurate predictions are difficult due to variation in patients' conditions, and unavoidable complications can occur.

4. Instructions for the Operation (Procedure/Test)
1) After patients completely recover from anesthesia in the recovery room, they are transferred to a patient room.
2) Bed rest is recommended for patients after surgery. When they go to the toilet or move around, they always should be supported by their caregivers to prevent them from falling.
3) To prevent complications such as atelectasis or pneumonia caused by anesthesia, patients are recommended to take deep breaths and cough a lot on the day of surgery.
4) If a patient is found not to be suitable for the robot to be used during robotic surgery, the surgery can be converted to open surgery.

5. Possibility of changing the procedure method or increasing the extent of the procedure
Please refer to items in No. 2 and No. 3.
During robotic surgery, the surgeon can convert the procedure to open surgery using the conventional approach depending on the progress of surgery and the patient's condition. However, if an urgent need to change the operative method or to broaden the extent of the operation arises (so urgent that there is no time to explain the situation to the patient and obtain consent from the patient), surgery will be performed first. Then, the reason for the change or addition to the surgical procedure and the result of surgery will be explained to the patient or the patient's surrogate.

6. Possible alternative interventions
In principle, the treatment of breast cancer is the complete surgical resection of the tumor. As another method of surgical dissection, patients can choose for the incision to be made on the skin above the breast without using a robot. Currently, robotic surgery is not included in benefit coverage in the Korean National Insurance. Further treatments for breast cancer include chemotherapy before and after surgery, hormone therapy, radiation therapy, and targeted therapy.

7. Possible consequences that can occur if the procedure is not performed
When breast cancer is not dissected, metastasis to other organs can occur, which can lead to death due to multiple organ failure.

8. Success rate (expected clinical prognosis)

Fig. 7-2. An example of the informed consent (English)

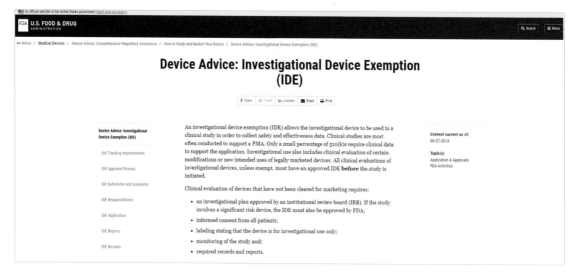

Fig. 7-3. The USFDA IDE website (https://www.fda.gov/medical-devices/how-study-and-market-your-device/investigational-device-exemption-ide)

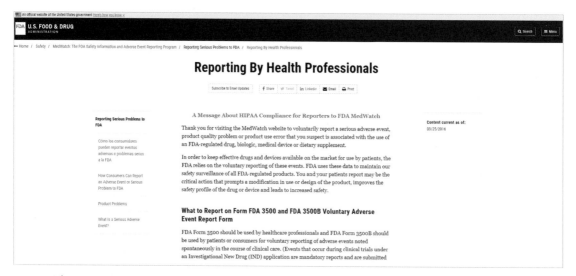

Fig. 7-4. The USFDA reporting website for health professionals (https://www.fda.gov/safety/reporting-serious-problems-fda/reporting-health-professionals)

Drawing of Incision at Ward

The brassiere line and the arm-covered areas of the axillary or lateral chest are drawn using a marker pen. A planned incision line is also drawn using a marker pen. Usually, the incision is located at the level of the nipple or the middle of the breast, between the mid and anterior axillary line (Fig. 7-5, 6).

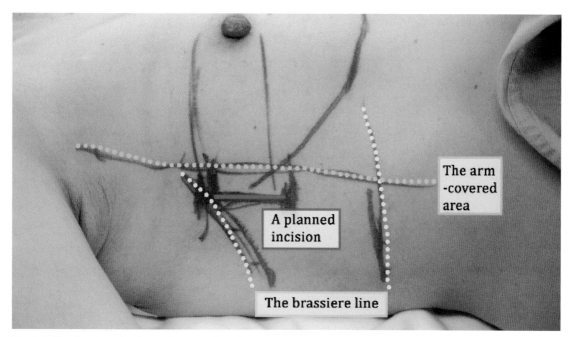

Fig. 7-5. The drawing of a planned incision for robotic mastectomy

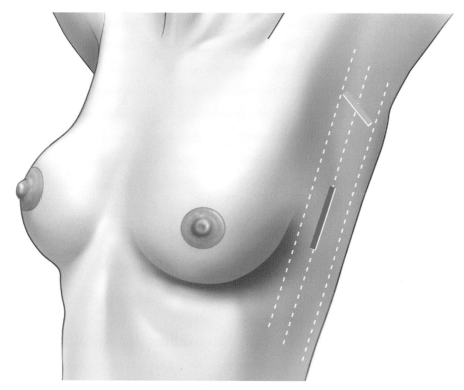

Fig. 7-6. Drawing of the incision. The green line indicates axillary incision. The red line indicates lateral incision in the mid-axillary line. The white dotted lines indicate anterior, mid, and posterior axillary lines.

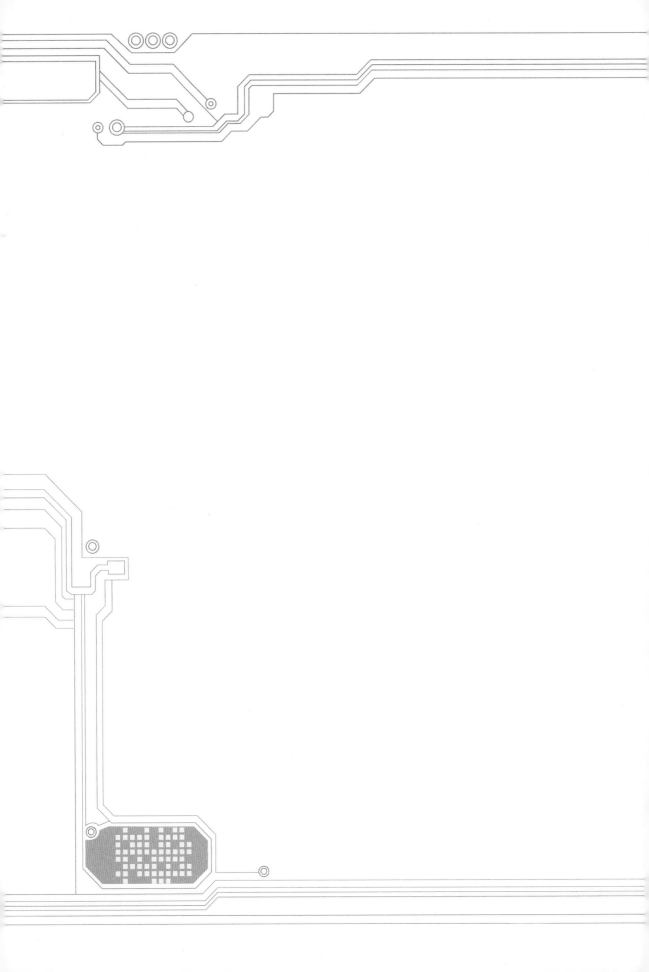

Robotic or Endoscopic Mastectomy

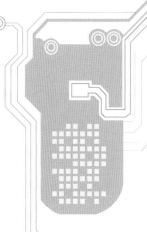

8. Gas-Inflated Robot-Assisted Nipple-Sparing Mastectomy

Hyung Seok Park

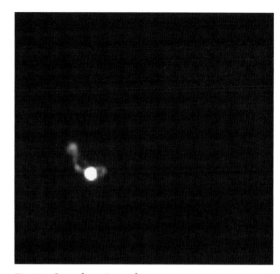

Fig. 8-1. Lymphangiography

0.5mCi Tc-99m phytate is injected into the periareolar area before surgery for a Breast lymphangiogram. A sentinel lymph node is noted in the right axilla (Fig. 8-1).

When you use conventional axillary incision, sentinel lymph node biopsy can easily be performed. However, collision can occur between the robotic arm placed near the armpit and the ipsilateral arm of the patient. For example, in RNSM for the right breast, the robotic arm with Prograsp forceps can frequently collide to the right arm of the patient, while for the left breast, the robotic arm with monopolar curved scissors can collide with the left arm. Extending the distance between the proximal and distal ring of the wound protector to 5-10 cm can be helpful to avoid collision with robotic arm and the patient's arm (Fig. 8-2b).

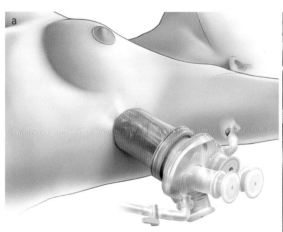
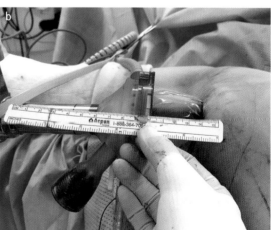

Fig. 8-2. Single port location

Therefore, I adopted Dr. Safarti's incision which is placed on the mid axillary line and level of the nipple or the middle of the breast for the gas-inflated RNSM (Fig. 7-6).

Sentinel lymph node biopsy through the incision at the mid axillary line is feasible because the incision is located near the armpit. Fiberoptic retractors and advanced energy devices can be helpful to perform sentinel lymph node biopsy or axillary lymph node dissection through this incision. This will be further discussed in the later section (55p, Sentinel lymph node dissection).

Position

After anesthesia, the patient is placed at the edge of the table. Sponges or pillow (Fig. 8-3) can be placed at the back of the patient to elevate the trunk.

Two types of arm boards, an anesthesia arm board with sheets instead of an arm board pad (Steris, Mentor, OH, USA, Fig. 8-4) and a raised arm board (Mizuho Medical Co., Tokyo, Japan, Fig. 8-5), are attached to the operation table (Fig. 8-6).

Surgical drapes are applied as per usual procedure (Fig. 8-7). The ipsilateral arm is separately draped to move up and down during the surgery.

The operation table is tilted to the contralateral side by 15-20 degrees. The operation table is elevated to the level of the surgeon's eyes when he/she is in the sitting position (Fig. 8-8).

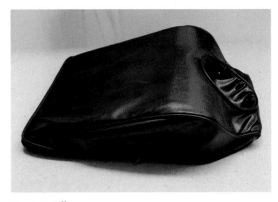

Fig. 8-3. Pillow

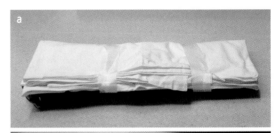

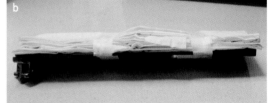

Fig. 8-4. Armboard

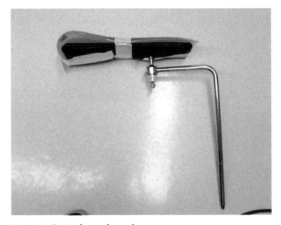

Fig. 8-5. Raised arm board

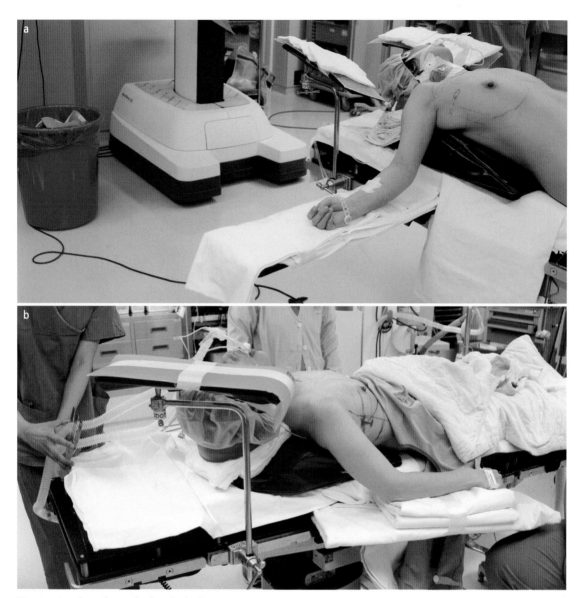

Fig. 8-6. Armboards attached to the bed

Table 8-1. Incision size and the breast weight

Specimen weight (g)	Final incision (cm)
≤ 200	3
200 < specimen ≤ 400	4
400 < specimen ≤ 600	5
600 < specimen ≤ 800	6
800 < specimen ≤ 1000	6~

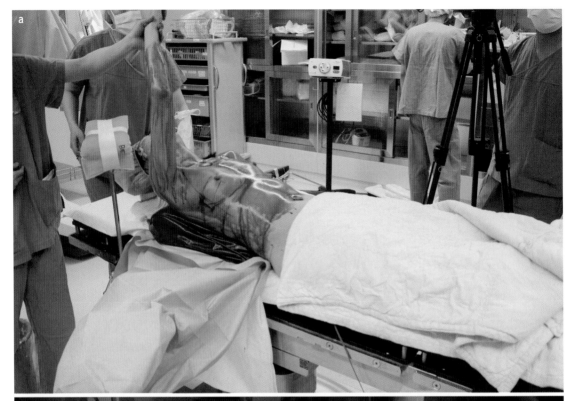

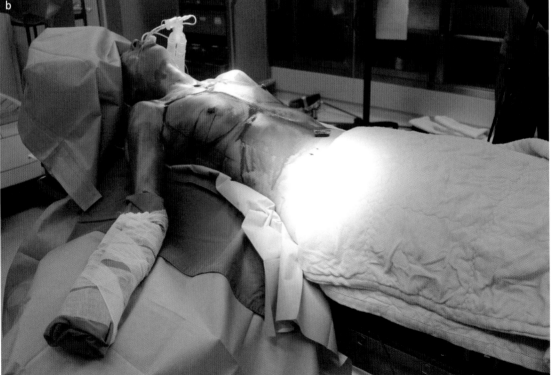

Fig. 8-7. **Arm drapping**

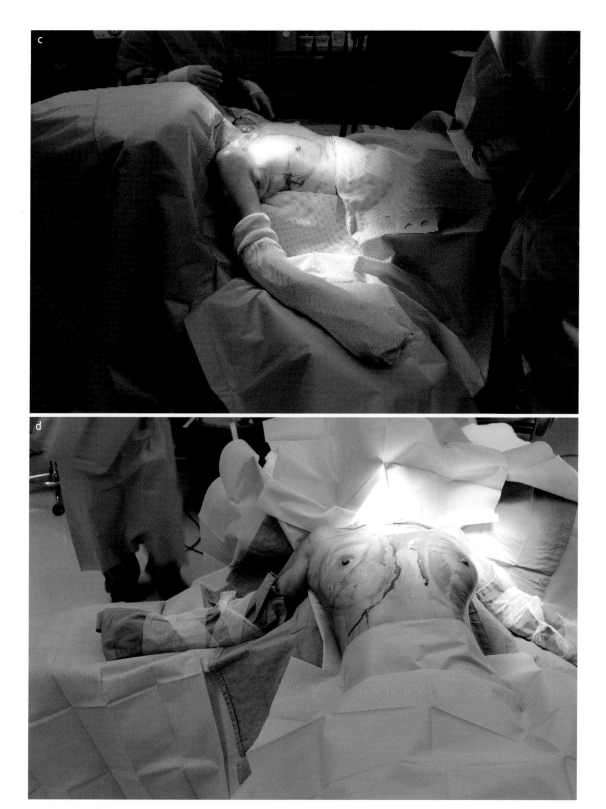

Fig. 8-7. Arm drapping

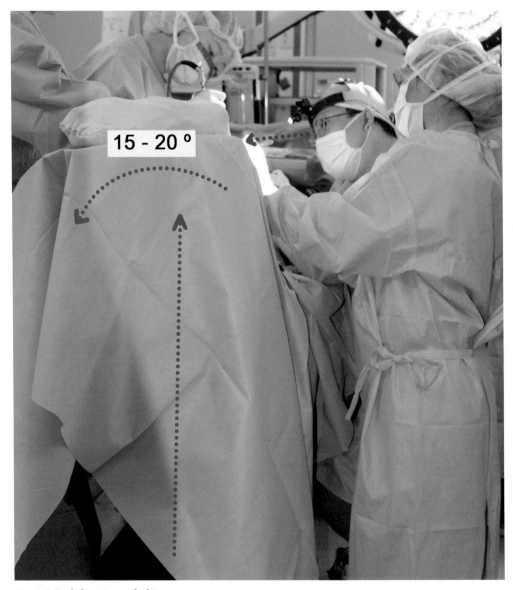

Fig. 8-8. Bed elevation and tilting

Incision design

The actual incision line is drawn using a marker pen. Incision size is made according to the breast volume/weight. The length of incision changes depending on the patient's position (Fig. 8-9).

The incision line is shortened when the arm position is lowered. Incision size is measured at the anatomical position, not the upright arm position. Even though approximately 3-4 cm is enough for less than 300 g of breast volume/weight for experienced surgeons, I recommend a 5-6 cm incision for beginners.

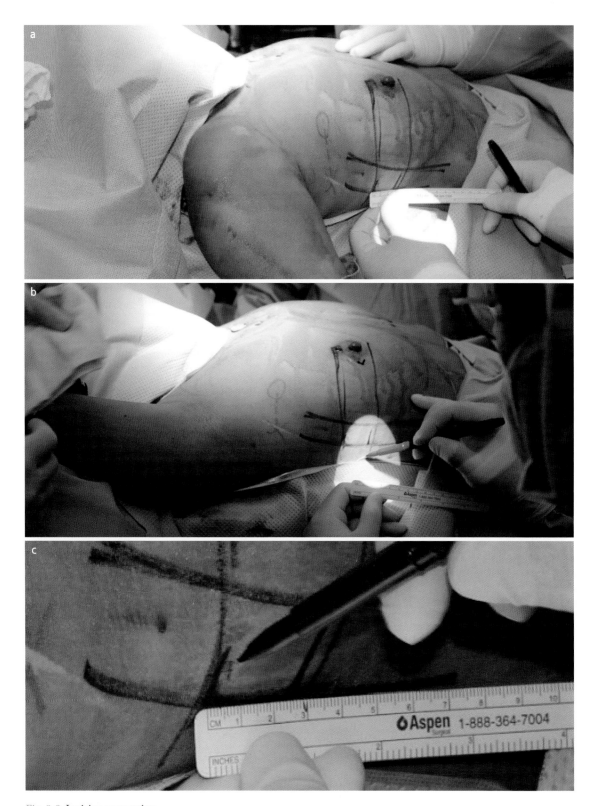

Fig. 8-9. Incision measuring

Marking of borders

Breast borders are lined using a marker pen (Fig. 8-10).

For sentinel lymph node biopsy and border-marking, blue dye is injected to periareolar area and breast borders (Fig. 8-11).

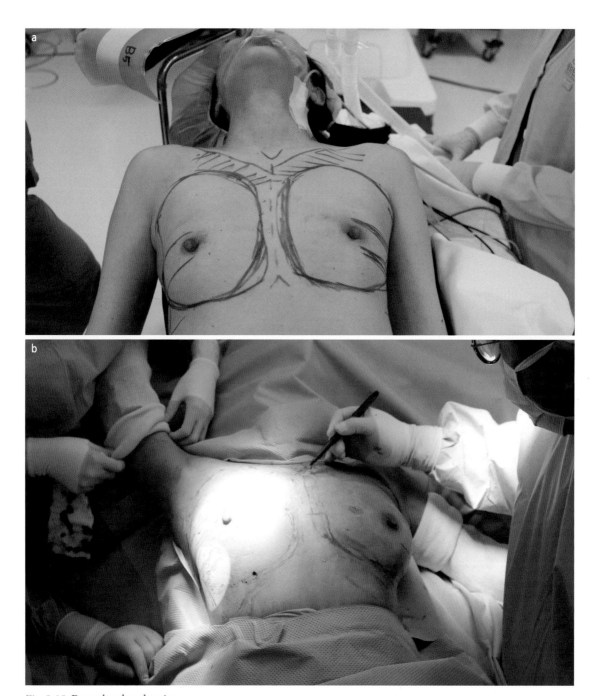

Fig. 8-10. Breast borders drawing

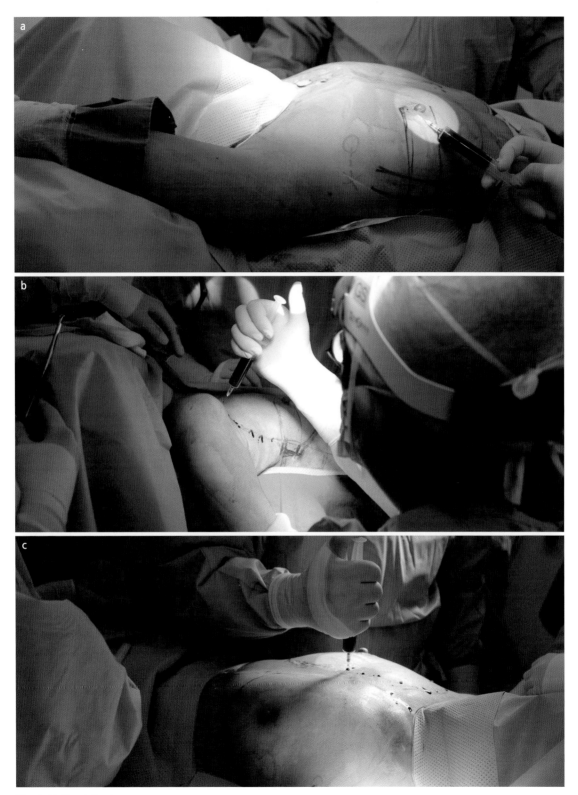

Fig. 8-11. Dye injection

A 28G short needle and syringe should be used for blue dye injection into the borders because a larger and longer needle can cause iatrogenic pneumothorax (Fig. 8-12, 13).

Blue dye injection for the breast border-marking is made into at least twelve points around the borders with 2-3 cm distance from each injection (Fig. 8-14).

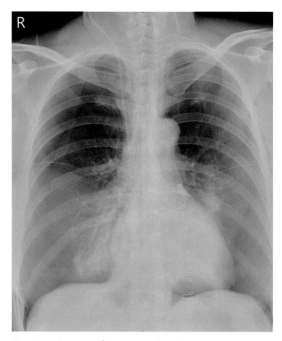

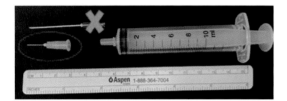

Fig. 8-12. Injection needle

Fig. 8-13. Pneumothorax

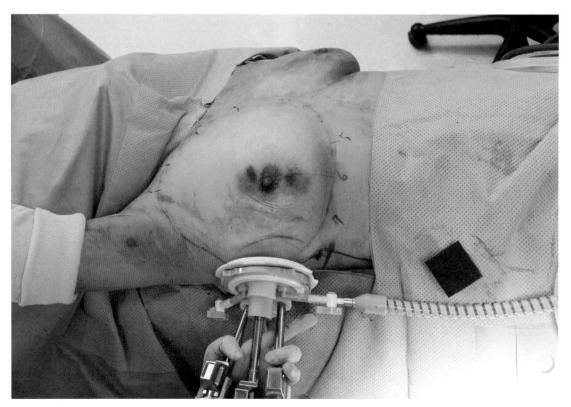

Fig. 8-14. Border marking by blue dye

Sentinel lymph node biopsy

After the incision is made, sentinel lymph node biopsy using electrocautery or advanced energy devices is performed. Senn or small Richardson retractors are applied to approach the axilla (Fig. 8-15).

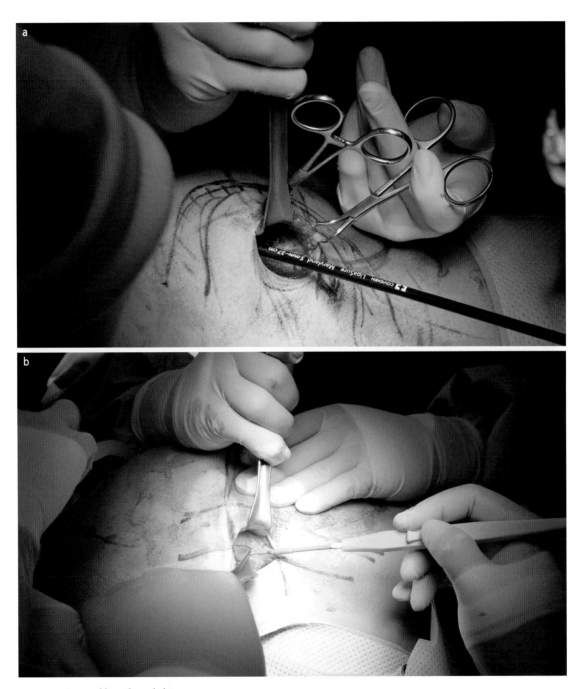

Fig. 8-15. Sentinel lymph node biopsy

When the clavicopectoral fascia is identified, a gamma probe is applied to detect the sentinel lymph nodes (Fig. 8-16).

Because of the longer distance between the incision and the axillary area than in conventional sentinel lymph node biopsy, advanced energy devices such as HARMONIC ACE® +7 Shears with Advanced Hemostasis

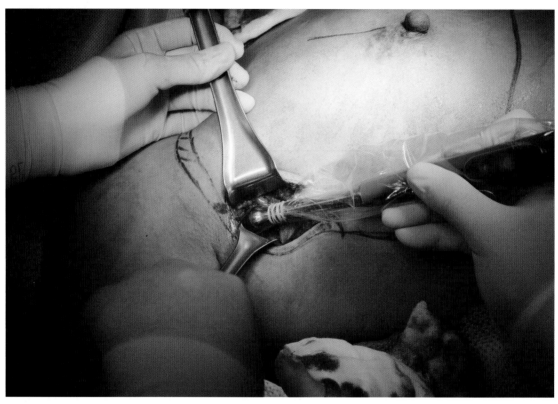

Fig. 8-16. Gamma probe

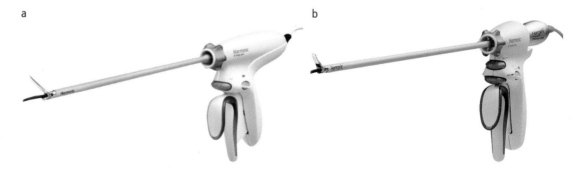

Fig. 8-17.
a. HARMONIC® HD 1000i Shears ©Ethicon, Inc. 2020
b. HARMONIC ACE® +7 Shears with Advanced Hemostasis ©Ethicon, Inc. 2020

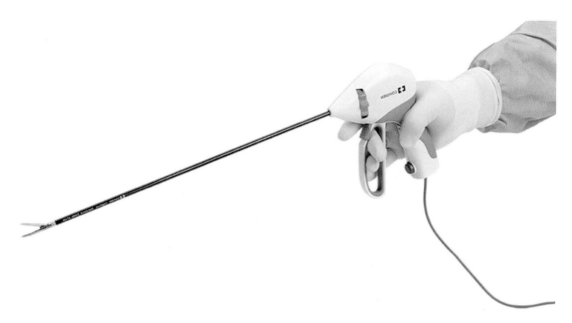

Fig. 8-18. Ligasure™ Maryland Jaw Open Sealer/Divider

(Ethicon Inc., Cornelia, GA, USA) and Ligasure™ Maryland Jaw Device with Nano-Coated Jaws (Medtronic, Minneapolis, MN, USA) can be used (Fig. 8-17, 18).

Advanced energy devices enable easier dissection and hemostasis for sentinel lymph node biopsy. Fiberoptic retractors can be used for better visualization of the operation field during sentinel lymph node biopsy (Fig. 8-19, 20).

Intraoperative frozen section can be used to identify the involvement of metastatic cells in

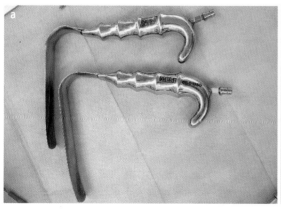
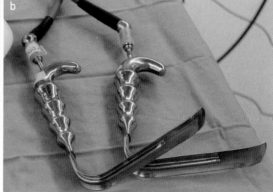

Fig. 8-19.
a. Fiberoptic retractors
b. Fiberoptic retractors with light source cable

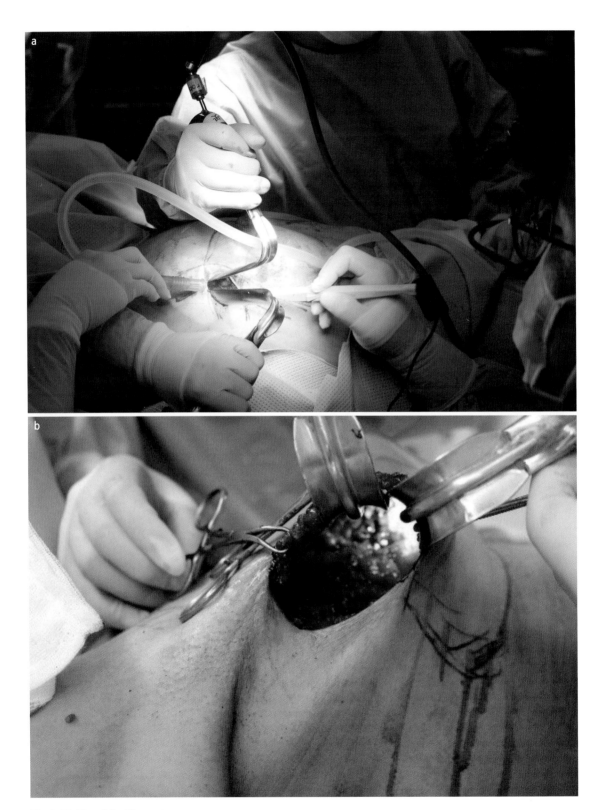

Fig. 8-20. Use of the fiberoptic retractors

sentinel lymph nodes. If metastasis is identified in a sentinel lymph node, conventional axillary lymph node dissection should be performed. Conventional axillary lymph node dissection can be done through the same axillary incision. It is sometimes helpful to make additional 1-2 cm extension of the incision for easier access to the axilla (Fig. 8-21).

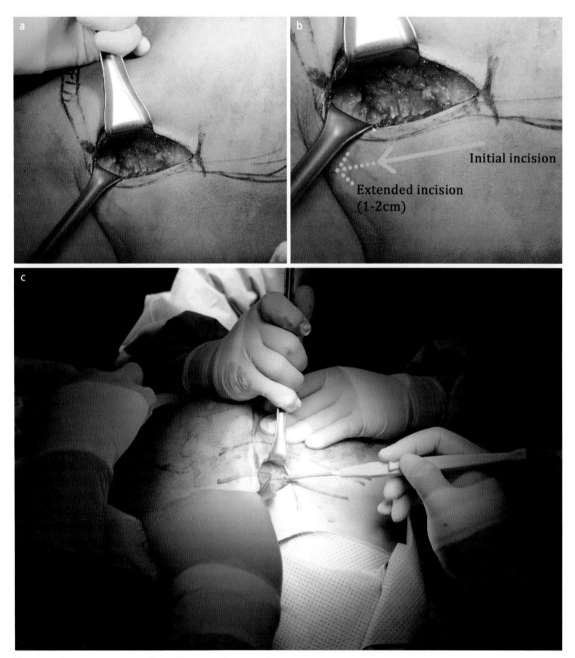

Fig. 8-21. Incision extension for axillary lymph nodes dissection

Creation of working space

After sentinel lymph node biopsy, working space should be made (Fig. 8-22). The size of the working space depends on the size of the ring of single port devices (Table 8-2).

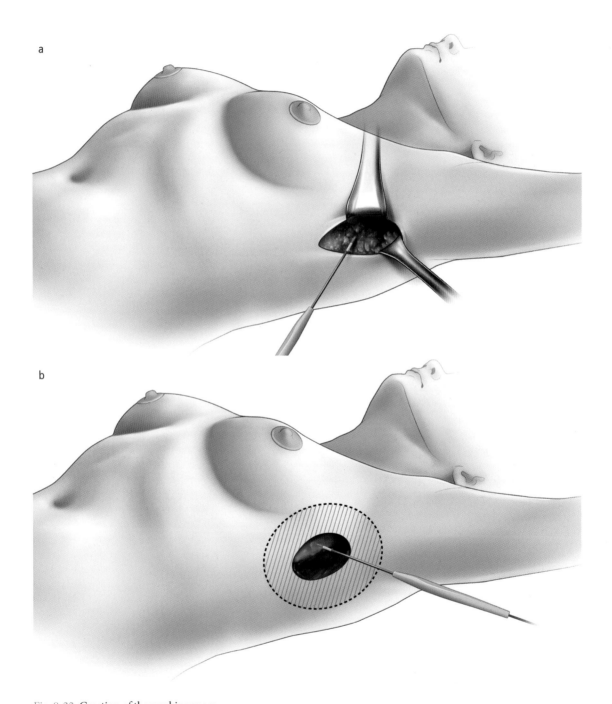

Fig. 8-22. Creation of the working space

Table 8-2. Various single port devices and the size of the working spaces

	Product	Docking state	The Largest Diameter of Wound Protectors
Manual glove port			7 cm
Oneport®			6 cm
OCTO™ port			9 cm
GelPoint®			7 cm
Lapsingle			N/A
UNI−PORT			9.2 cm

Estimated area of the working space is marked with the ring using a marker pen (Fig. 8-23).

For example, when you use OCTO™port (Jireh Korea Rapha, Seoul, Korea) as a single port device for robotic mastectomy, 2.5-3.0 cm of incision size and 4.0-5.0 cm diameter of the semicircular working space are sufficient.

When you use OCTO™Port (DalimsurgNET Co., Ltd., Seoul, Korea), 3.0-5.0 cm of incision size and 5.0-7.0 cm diameter of the semicircular working space are needed. If you make a larger incision than recommended, air leaking beside the ring will occur, and this will disturb the procedure. If air leaks despite using the appropriate incision size, 1-2 sutures at the

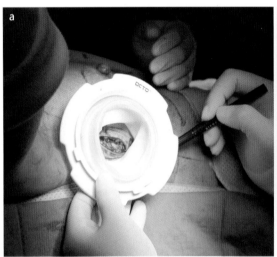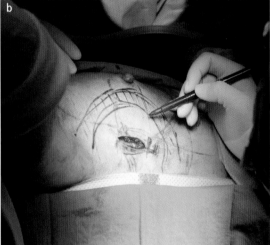

Fig. 8-23. Drawing of the working space

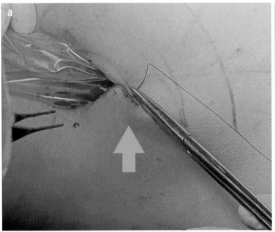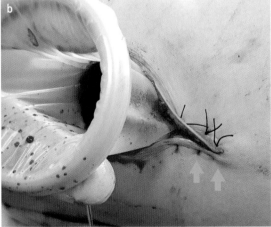

Fig. 8-24. Suture for preventing air leak

edge of the incision may reduce the leaking (Fig. 8-24).

The working space of the superficial layer of the superficial fascia is made using a monopolar electrocautery by the line that you drew as the estimated area of the working space (Fig. 8-25).

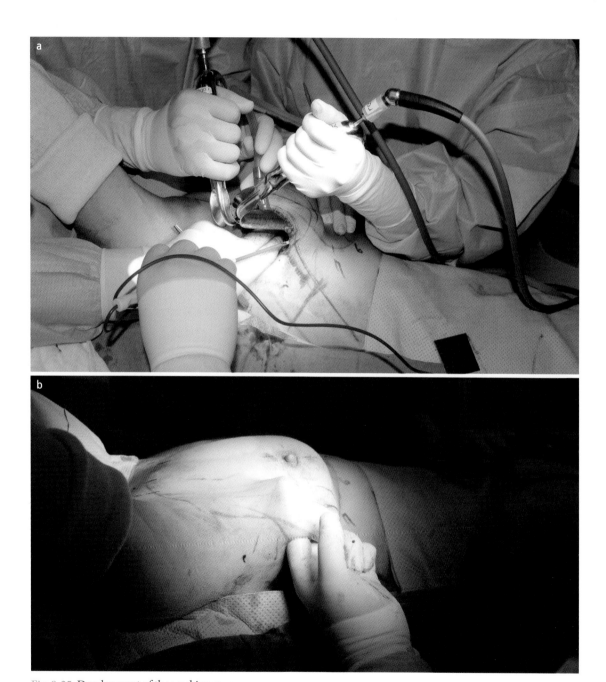

Fig. 8-25. Development of the working space

Retromammary space dissection

Retromammary space dissection to the breast borders marked by the blue dye can be manually performed using fiberoptic retractors, monopolar electrocautery, and/or advanced energy devices (Fig. 8-26).

I prefer this method. The more you dissect manually, the more you can reduce the operation time. Caution should be taken to identify the lateral border of the pectoral major muscle (Fig. 8-27).

It is a bit difficult to distinguish the interpectoral and retromammary spaces even in the manual dissection via the small lateral incision. The lateral border of the pectoral major muscle including upper and lower lateral borders, 7-11 o'clock direction for right breast and 1-5 o'clock direction for left breast, should be fully dissected as much as possible in the manual dissection (Fig. 8-28).

You can also dissect the retromammary space using the robotic system after docking.

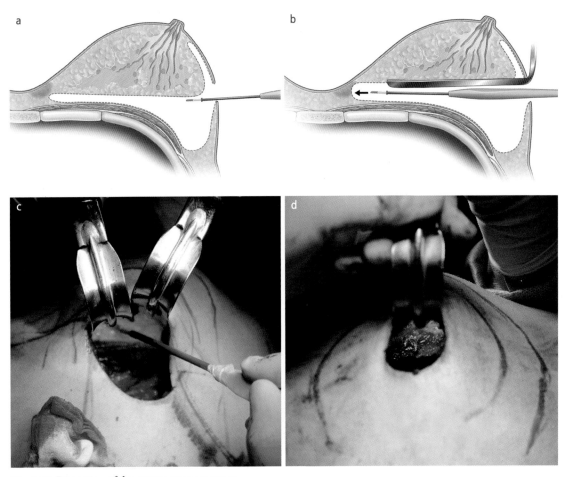

Fig. 8-26. Dissection of the retromammary space

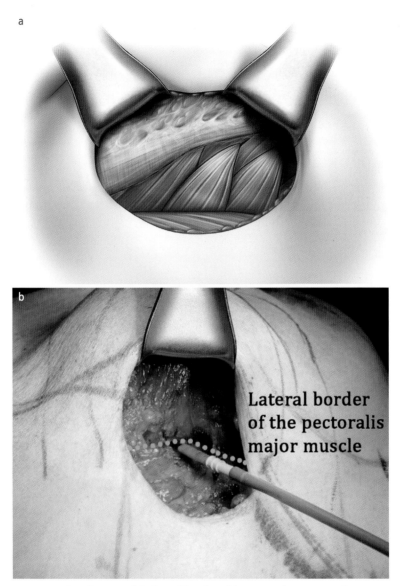

Fig. 8-27. Identification of the lateral border of the pectoral major muscle

However, it may consume a longer operation time because redundant breast parenchyma can often interfere with visualization of the field. You should be careful of bleeding from perforator vessels during the retromammary space dissection. However, this bleeding can be controlled using a long shaft or Maryland -type of advanced energy devices (Fig. 8-29).

Injection of the tumescent solution

Injection of the tumescent solution containing normal saline 1000 cc, lidocaine 1% (200 mg/V), and epinephrine 1 mg/A to the superficial layer of the superficial fascia is

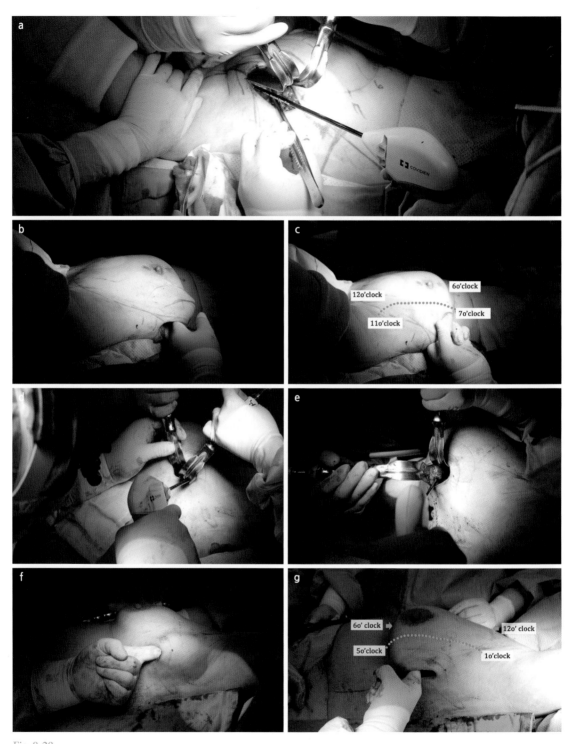

Fig. 8-28.
a. The range of the dissection of the lateral border of the pectoral major muscle
b. The lower range of the dissection of the lateral border of the pectoral major muscle
c. The upper range of the dissection of the lateral border of the pectoral major muscle
d-g. The range of the dissection of the lateral border of the pectoral major muscle

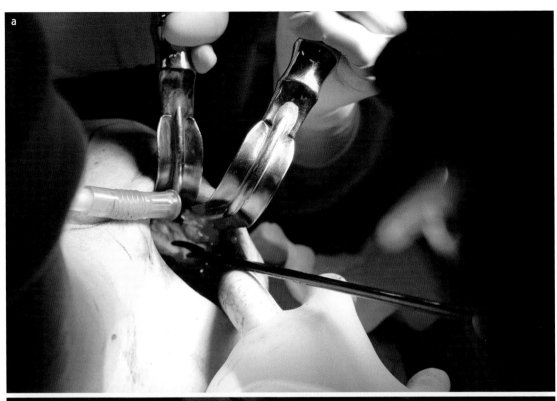

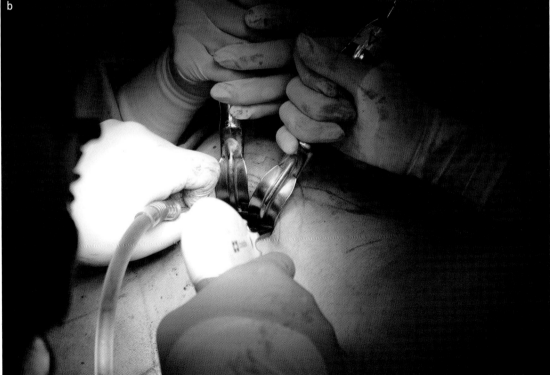

Fig. 8-29. Bleeding Control using Harmonic

applied for hydrodissection (Fig. 8-30).

Long 18G needles and 50 cc disposable syringes are used to deliver the injection of the tumescent solution (Fig. 8-31-a~c). The Veress needle can be utilized for the injection of the tumescent solution without skin puncture because the length of the Veress needle is long enough to approach to the medial border of the breast from the incision (Fig. 8-31-d~f).

The volume of the injected tumescent solution depends on the size of the breast. I recommend about 200-300 cc for small sized

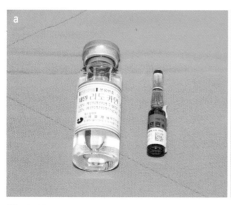
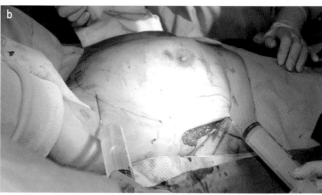

Fig. 8-30.
a. Lidocaine 1% and epinephrine 1 mg for 1 L tumescent solution
b. Injection of the tumescent solution

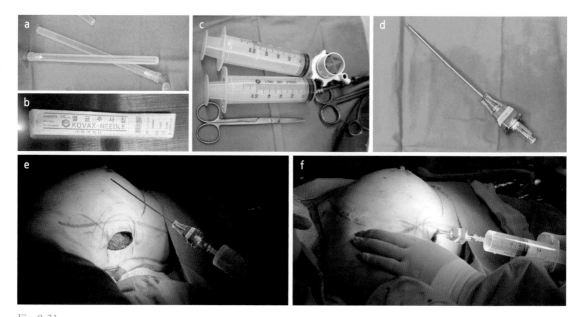

Fig. 8-31.
a-c. Needles and syringes for the injection of the tumescent solution
d. the Veress needle
e-f. Tumescent injection using the Veress needle

breasts, 300 cc for medium sized breasts, and 300–400 cc for large sized breasts. Using fine Metzenbaum scissors or vascular tunneler, subcutaneous tunneling to the whole breast is achieved. The distance interval between tunnels is about 2–3 cm (Fig. 8-32).

It is beneficial to achieve an appropriate subcutaneous tunneling for better visualization of the operation field by air extension to the

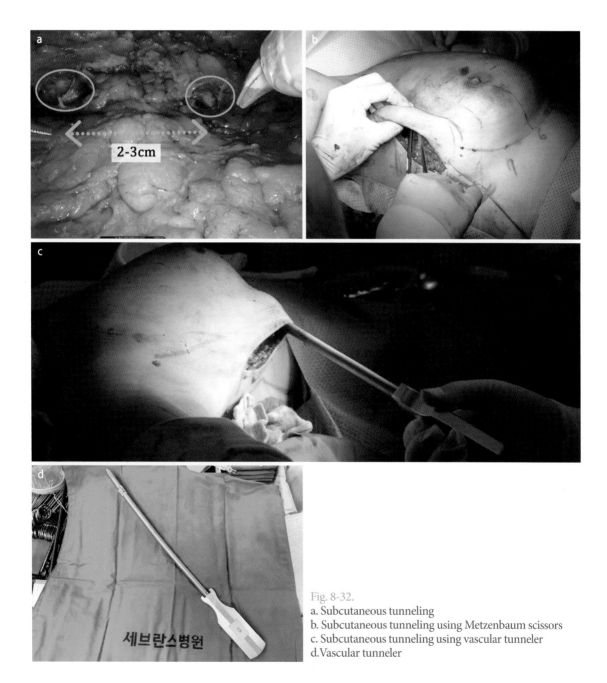

Fig. 8-32.
a. Subcutaneous tunneling
b. Subcutaneous tunneling using Metzenbaum scissors
c. Subcutaneous tunneling using vascular tunneler
d. Vascular tunneler

whole subcutaneous tissue of the breast. After tunneling, you can genthly roll the gauze or sponge along the breast to push the remaining fluid of the injected tumescent solution out to the incision site (Fig. 8-33).

Attachment of single port device

Before attaching a single port device, the remaining gauze or sponge in the working space should be removed through incision. The single port device is attached to the incision site. There are various single port devices (Table 8-2). OCTO™port is one of the single port devices for robotic mastectomy. Here is the detailed process of the attachment of OCTO™port (Fig. 8-34).

Finger palpation to the working space through the ring of the single port device is beneficial to understand the appropriate position of the internal ring and the breast parenchyma. Be cautious not to overlap the internal ring and the breast parenchyma (Fig. 8-35). Should that be the case, you will see the retromammary space instead of the subcutaneous space, as well as tunnels that were made during the working space dissection and subcutaneous tunneling.

Hanging suture for pulling of nipple-areolar complex

A one-point hanging suture using 3-0 silk is applied to pull up the nipple-areolar complex for safer dissection during the console procedure (Fig. 8-36). Mosquito clamps hold the hanging suture.

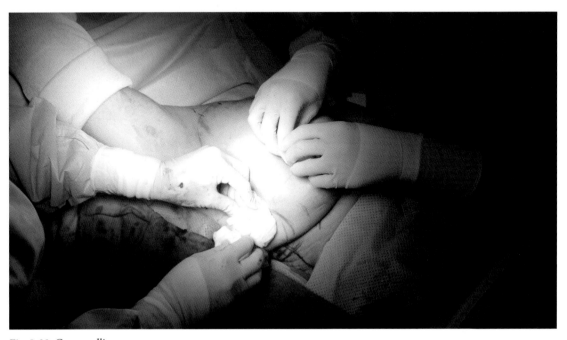

Fig. 8-33. Gauze rolling

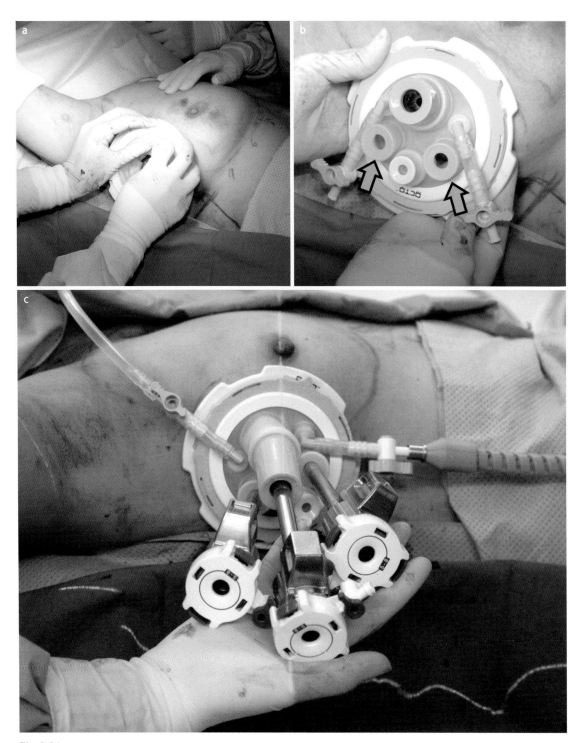

Fig. 8-34.

a. OCTO™port attachment: wound protector is inserted into the incision

b. OCTO™port attachment: single port device is connected to wound protector. Two white plastic rings of the 5 mm-lumens are removed for 8 mm-robotic cannulas.

c. OCTO™port attachment: cannulas are inserted into the lumens

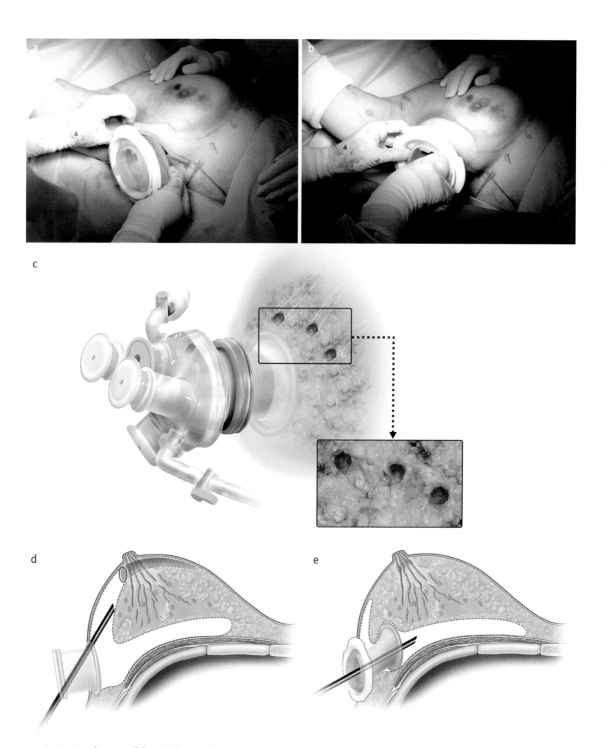

Fig. 8-35. Attachment of the single port device
a. Insertion of a wound protector of a single port device
b. Identification of the appropriate position of the internal ring and the breast parenchyma
c. Internal view of the subcutaneous tunneling
d. Appropriate position of the internal ring of the wound protector and camera
e. Inappropriate position of the internal ring of the wound protector and camera

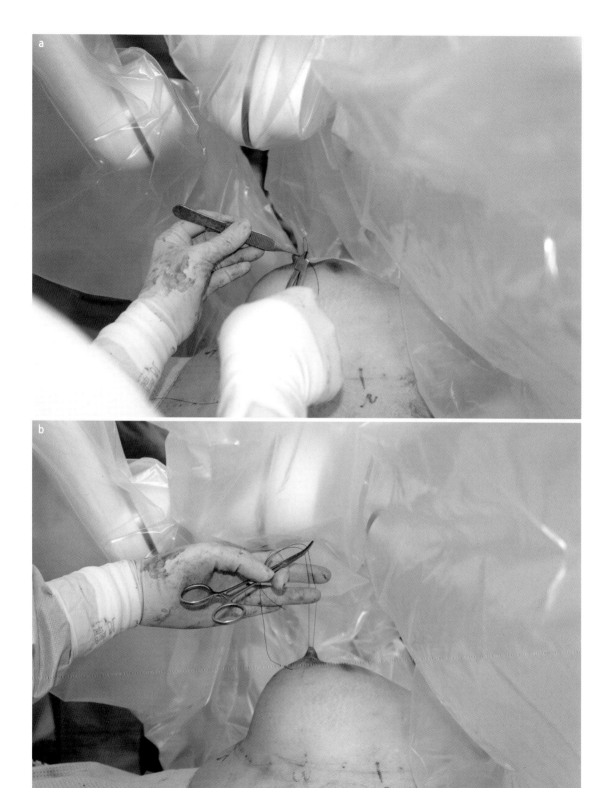

Fig. 8-36. Pulling of nipple-areolar complex

Docking

A patient cart is placed at the counter side of the breast or by the patient's head side (Fig. 8-37). The level of the operating table should be put to the lowest level to avoid inflicting any injury on the patient's head and trunk with the

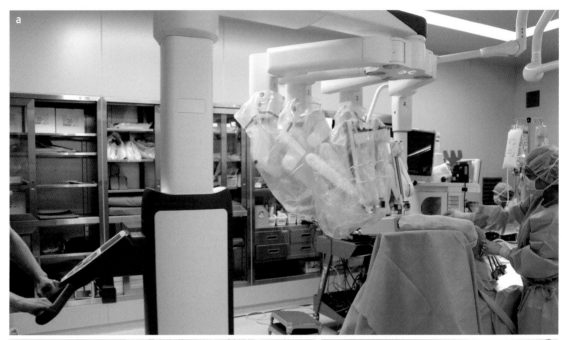

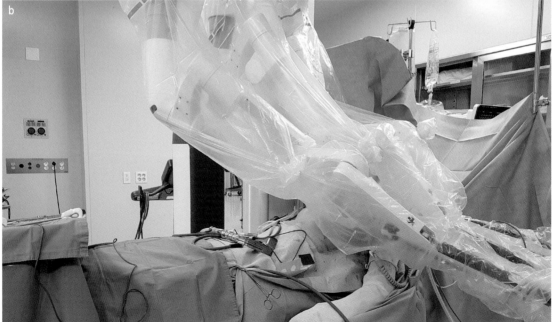

Fig. 8-37. The location of the patient cart - the contralateral side of the ipsilateral breast

robotic arms.

The patient cart is advanced to the ipsilateral breast. The robotic arms are located above the breast (Fig. 8-38).

The green laser cross point is placed on the remote center of the camera cannula (Fig. 8-39).

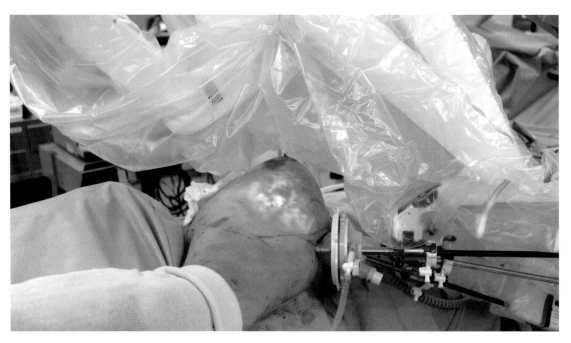

Fig. 8-38. The robotic arms above the breast

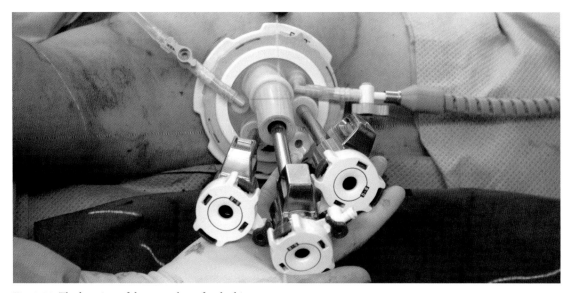

Fig. 8-39. The location of the green laser for docking

The transverse green laser line is placed at the level of the nipple. The cannulas are inserted into the right and the left entry of the single port device (Fig. 8-40).

Robotic arms are attached to each cannula. First, the 30-degree robotic camera is placed

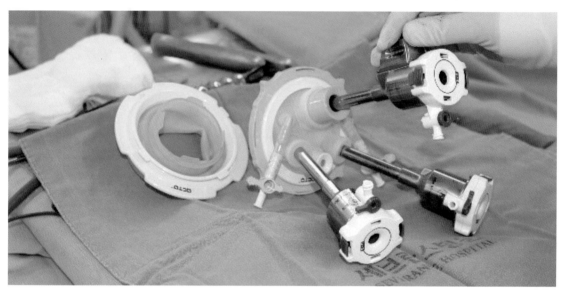

Fig. 8-40. The cannulas are inserted into the single port device

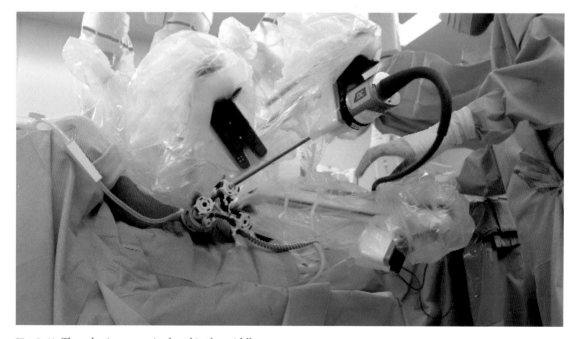

Fig. 8-41. The robotic camera is placed in the middle arm

facing up in the middle arm (Fig. 8-41).

Then, Prograsp forceps and monopolar curved scissors are inserted into the left and right arms, respectively (Fig. 8-42, 43).

The instruments, including the Prograsp forceps, camera, and monopolar curved

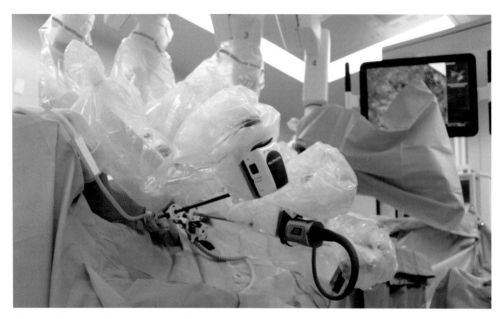

Fig. 8-42. Prograsp forceps are inserted into the left arm

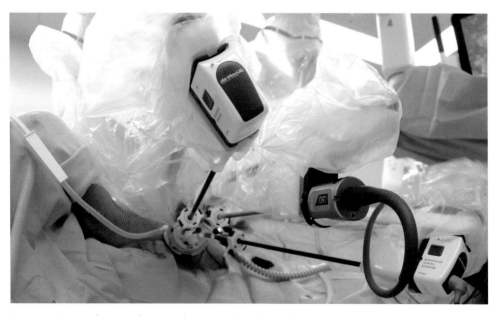

Fig. 8-43. Monopolar curved scissors are inserted into the right arm

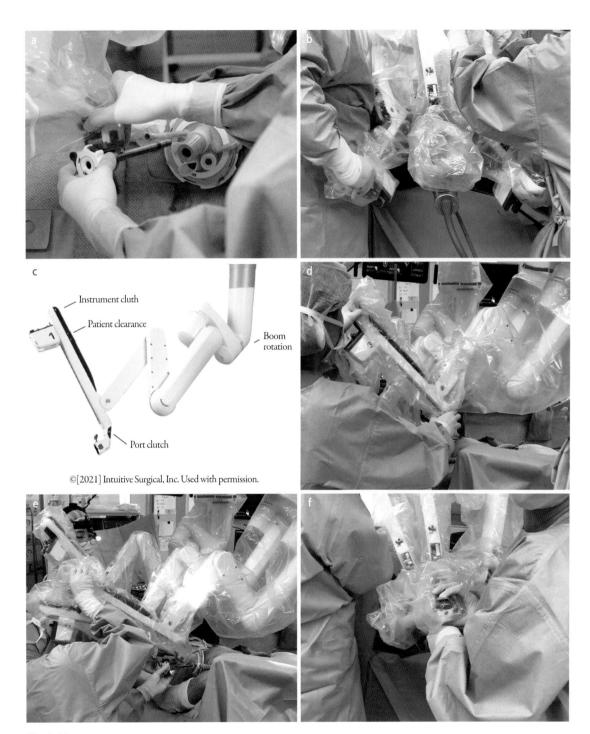

Fig. 8-44.
a. Docking with clutch control using a cannula mount lever
b. Docking with clutch control using the instrument clutch
c. Buttons on arms to initiate movement[1]
d, e. Clutch control using instrument and port clutches
f. Clutch control using a instrument clutch

Instrument cluth
Patient clearance
Boom rotation
Port clutch

©[2021] Intuitive Surgical, Inc. Used with permission.

scissors should be moved into the working space using arm and port clutches (Fig. 8-44).

If you complete the docking, you will see the tunnels of the subcutaneous tissue (Fig. 8-45).

The positions of the instruments are placed in a triangular position (Fig. 8-46).

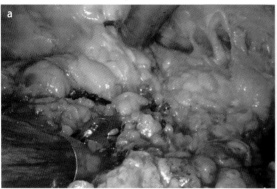
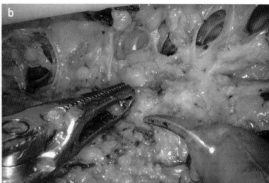

Fig. 8-45. The tunnels of the subcutaneous tissue

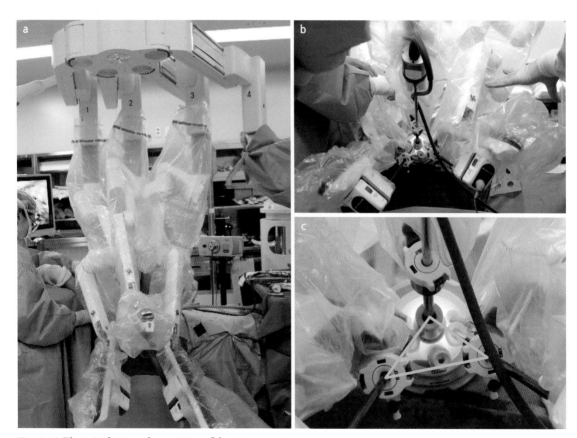

Fig. 8-46. The initial triangular position of the instruments

Console

Before the console procedure, you can adjust the console ergonomics or load the pre-setting of the console ergonomics (Fig. 8-47).

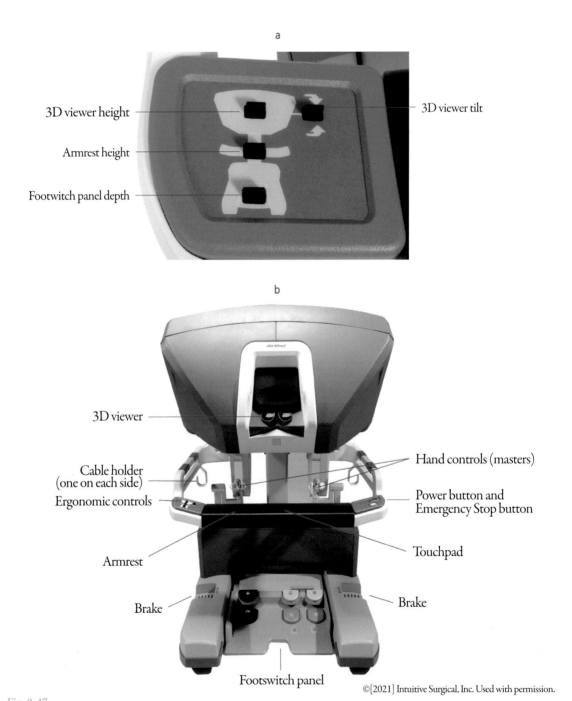

a

3D viewer height — 3D viewer tilt

Armrest height

Footwitch panel depth

b

3D viewer

Cable holder (one on each side) — Hand controls (masters)

Ergonomic controls — Power button and Emergency Stop button

Armrest — Touchpad

Brake — Brake

Footswitch panel

©[2021] Intuitive Surgical, Inc. Used with permission.

Fig. 8-47.
a. Ergonomic controls in the Left-side
b. Parts of the surgeon console

You can see the triangular position of the instruments (Fig. 8-46). I prefer to have the dissection toward the nipple-areolar complex as the first step of the procedure to reduce the operation time because the frozen section of the nipple takes 20-30 minutes. The dissection of the nipple-areolar complex should be cautiously performed to avoid tearing of the skin or nipple-areolar complex.

I prefer to dissect and obtain nipple core to evaluate the involvement of the tumor with counter-retraction using the prograsp forceps and the cutting mode of the electrocautery or by slightly cutting using MCS (Fig. 8-48).

The first assistant prepares additional endoscopic forceps and inserts them into the third entry of the single port device to take the nipple core out for the frozen section (Fig. 8-49).

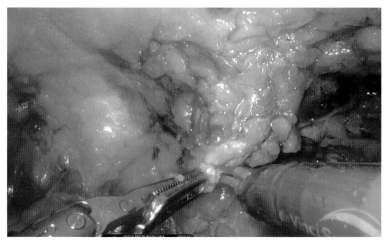

Fig. 8-48. Obtaining nipple core

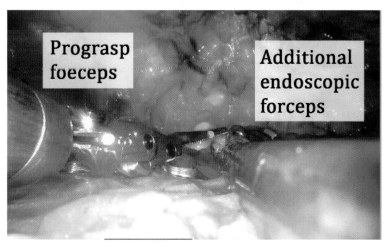

Fig. 8-49. Retrieval of nipple core

The next step is the dissection of the medial, upper, and lower parts of the subcutaneous tissue along with the tunnels. The tunneling that you made before the docking helps you to identify dissection plane more easily (Fig. 8-50).

You may have some difficulties visualizing the tunneling because of the blind spot made by the 30-degree-up camera at some point, which usually appears after the dissection of NAC. When that happens, the camera position should be changed to 30-degree-down. Before you change the camera position, move the camera

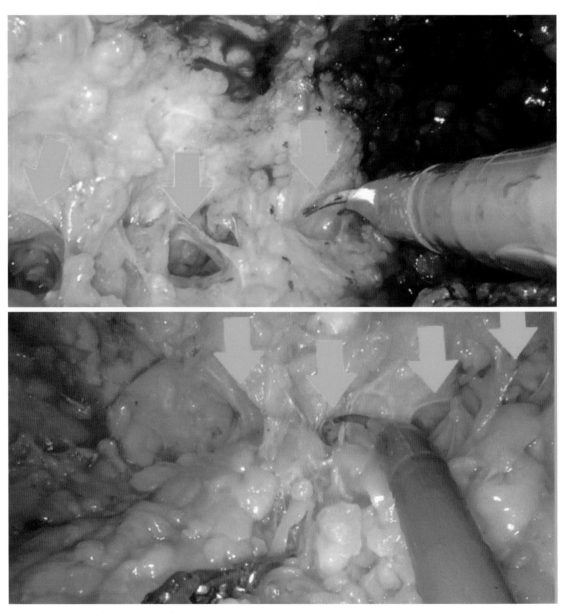

Fig. 8-50. Tunnels of subcutaneous layer

as near as possible to the superficial layer to avoid the vision from getting blurred(Fig. 8-51b) because the breast parenchyma touches the camera lense (Fig. 8-51a).

The remaining dissection toward the upper, inner, and lower borders should be made until the injected blue dye is visualized. If you are not familiar with the blue dye injection to the borders, the assistant can advise the anatomical location of the borders with gentle palpation on them during the procedure (Fig. 8-52).

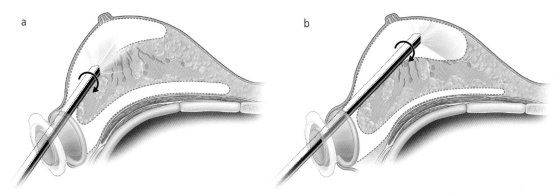

Fig. 8-51. The change of the camera position

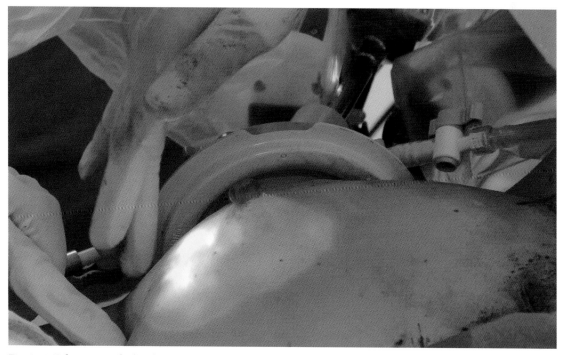

Fig. 8-52. Palpation on the borders

Tips for easier approach to the dissection plane of the medial border and for reducing collision of robotic arms.

When you dissect the medial area of the breast, it may be difficult to approach this part by MCS because of the convex shape of the dome of the breast parenchyma. To make it easier to approach this part, I prefer to dissect the retromammary space as much as possible before docking. In addition, you should remember the following three tips after docking. First, ask the assistant to move MCS down 1-2 cm using port or arm clutches of the robotic arms in the patient cart (Fig. 8-53a). Second, counter-retract the medial part of the breast tissue using Prograsp forceps (Fig. 8-53b). Third, ask the assistant to adjust the distance between robotic arms to avoid collisions (Fig. 8-53c). Fourth, when you dissect the mediosuperior border of the breast, cross the MCS underneath the Prograsp to make it easier to counter-retract and dissect the tissue, Park's High Grasper and Low Scissors (HiGLoS) maneuver (Fig. 8-53d).

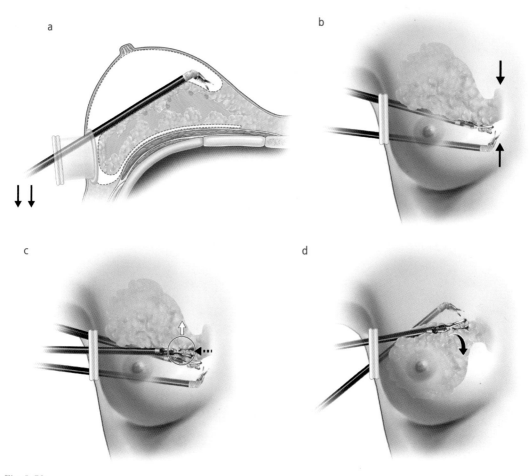

Fig. 8-53.
a. The modification of the location of MCS
b. The counter retraction of the breast parenchyma using Prograsp forceps
c. The retraction by an assistant
d. Park's High Grasper and Low Scissors (HiGLoS) maneuver

Specimen retrieval

After complete detachment of the breast parenchyma, the operator should confirm that adequate hemostasis has been achieved with careful inspection using 30-degree camera up and down. The docking is released from the single port device. It is nearly impossible to retrieve the breast tissue through an incision less than 3cm in length. Therefore, in most cases, an additional 1-2 cm extension of the incision is necessary to retrieve the breast tissue. Additional extension of the incision

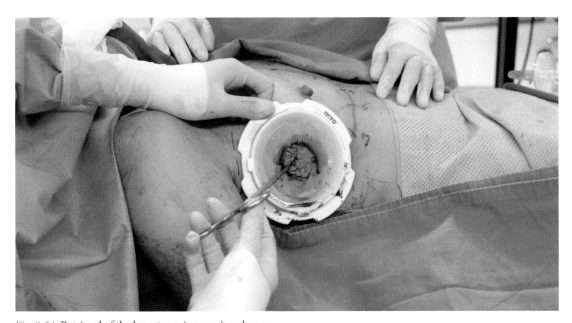

Fig. 8-54. Retrieval of the breast specimen using clamps

depends on the size of initial incisions and breast volumes/weights. Longer initial incisions, 3-6 cm, can be made using OCTO™port, while only 2.5-3 cm incisions can be applied for Oneport®. If you use OCTO™port and make an incision longer than 4 cm for robotic mastectomy, you can retrieve breast specimens larger than 250g. Table 8-1 shows retrieved breast weight and the incision size (Table 8-1). You can retrieve the breast tissue through the wound protector or the ring of the single port device (Fig. 8-54), but this depends on incision size and breast volume/weight.

After the retrieval of the specimen

After the retrieval of the breast tissue, you should inspect the surgical margins of the breast tissue. The surgical margins should be carefully evaluated to confirm grossly safe margins using inspection and palpation. Frozen section for the surgical margins can be applied if there is a suspicious lesion. The operator also can palpate the subcutaneous flap. When you find that the subcutaneous flap is thicker than 5 mm or that there is tumor involvement in the superficial margins, you can dissect additional subcutaneous flaps using Metzenbaum scissors or electrocautery to achieve oncologic safety.

Irrigation using normal saline is applied. The pocket of the prepectoral space can be inspected with fiberoptic retractors to find hidden bleeding sites. After completion of the procedure, immediate breast reconstruction begins.

9. Gasless Robot-Assisted Nipple-Sparing Mastectomy

Hyung Seok Park

Position

The position of the patient in the gasless robot-assisted Nipple-Sparing mastectomy is the same as with the gas-inflated robot-assisted Nipple-Sparing mastectomy (Fig. 8-3~8).

Incision design

A longer incision is needed in the gasless technique compared to the gas technique because the gasless technique needs insertion of a self-retractor into the working space. A 4-6 cm vertical skin incision is made in the anterior axillary line.

Marking of borders and sentinel lymph node biopsy

Marking of borders and sentinel lymph node biopsy are performed with the same methods as in the gas-inflated robot-assisted Nipple-Sparing mastectomy (Fig. 8-11~21).

Creation of working space

After the sentinel lymph node biopsy, a subcutaneous flap dissection toward the nipple-areolar complex is prepared through the incision using electrocautery. Undermining of a subcutaneous flap to the nipple-areolar complex from the axilla should be performed as much as possible to insert a self-retractor, the Chung's retractor (Fig. 9-1) and to reduce operation time in console. You should balance between manual and robotic dissection. Manual dissection is difficult to perform particularly in the medial part of the breast, but it reduces operation time. Robotic dissection is easier to perform, but it takes a longer time.

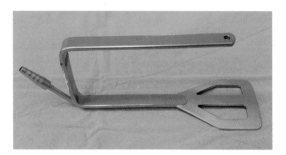

Fig. 9-1. A self-retractor, the Chung's retractor

Dissection of nipple-areolar complex

You can manually dissect the nipple-areolar complex through the 4-6 cm axillary incision. This is one of the main differences between my gas and gasless techniques. The longer incision of the gasless technique enables surgeons to obtain the tissue beneath the nipple manually (Fig. 9-2).

The assistant can flip the nipple with their finger to expose the retroareolar tissue, thus allowing the operator to resect the retroareolar

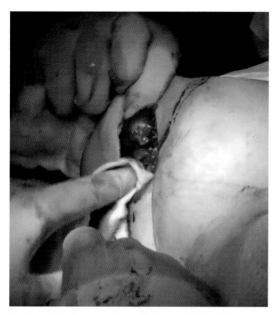

Fig. 9-2. Nipple core is identified via axilla incision before robot docking

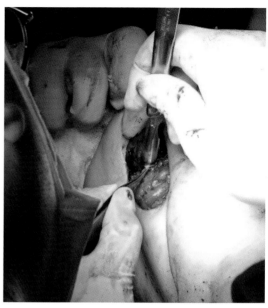

Fig. 9-3. Retroareolar tissue resection before docking

tissue using a scalpel with counter-retraction through Edson forceps (Fig. 9-3).

This is the so-called apple coring technique.[1] All breast tissue beneath the nipple have to be resected up to the dermis.[1] An intraoperative frozen section is performed to confirm a negative tumor margin.

One of the main advantages of this approach is that you can confirm involvement of tumor cells in the nipple-areolar complex before robot docking. It may be beneficial for patients with equivocal findings of nipple-areolar complex involvement in pre-operative evaluations. If you identify the nipple-areolar complex involvement in the frozen section, you should sacrifice the nipple and can perform skin-sparing mastectomy through a circumareolar incision instead of

RNSM. Because robot docking incurs cost regardless of the use of the robotic surgical systems, identifying nipple-areolar complex involvement before docking may be helpful.

You can offer patients the option of foregoing the use of robotic surgical systems in the situation that the nipple-areolar complex must be sacrificed according to the result of the intraoperative frozen section.

For example, one of my patients had equivocal findings of nipple-areolar complex involvement in the pre-operative evaluation (Fig. 9-4).

In this case, I prepared the gasless technique and manually dissected the tissue beneath the nipple-areolar complex. The frozen section revealed tumor involvement in the tissue, thus the nipple-areolar complex was

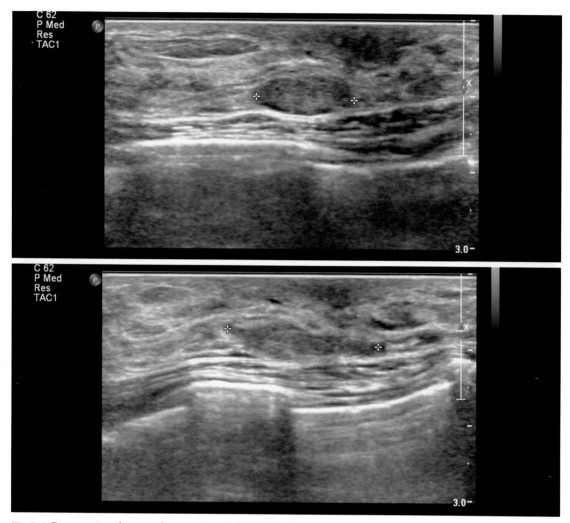

Fig. 9-4. Preoperative ultrasound in a patient with NAC involvement

sacrificed. Skin-sparing mastectomy using a circumareolar incision was performed. The cost for the use of robotic surgical systems is minimized using this method.

Retromammary space dissection

Retromammary tissue is dissected through a similar method in the gas technique. You can use fiberoptic retractors or the Chung's retractor to lift up the breast parenchyma (Fig. 9-5).

Retromammary space dissection can be performed till the injected blue dye is visualized in the breast borders (Fig. 9-6).

Injection of the tumescent solution

Tumescent solution is injected in the same manner as the gas technique.

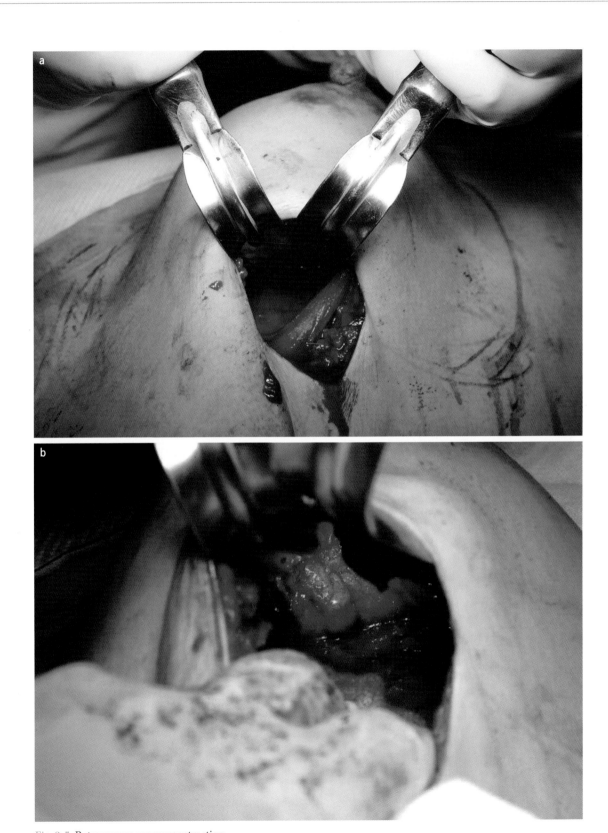

Fig. 9-5. Retromammary space retraction

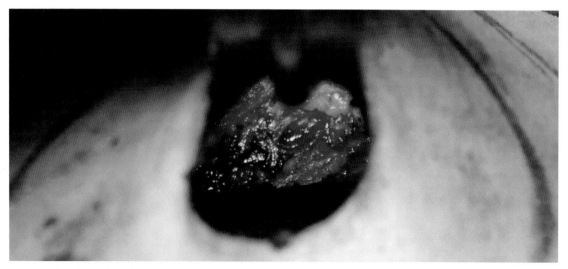

Fig. 9-6. Blue dye is identified via the incision after retromammary space dissection

Application of the self-retractor

The Chung's self-retractor consists of 6 parts
(Fig. 9-7):

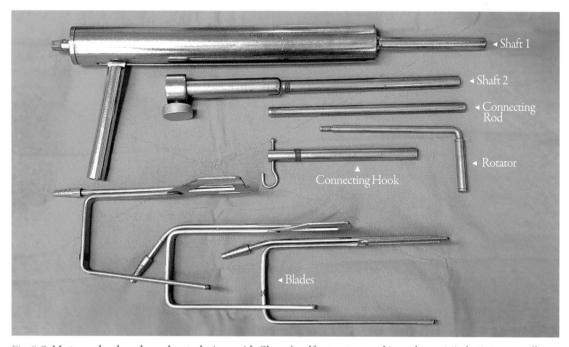

Fig. 9-7. My team developed a gasless technique with Chung's self-retractor, used in endoscopic/robotic trans-axillary thyroidectomy, for mastectomy using robotic surgical systems

Docking

A dual-channel 30-degree down camera is placed on the central arm. Fenestrated bipolar forceps or ProGrasp forceps and a permanent cautery spatula or monopolar curved scissors are placed on either side of the camera. For the gasless technique, additional Fenestrated bipolar forceps or ProGrasp forceps can be mounted on the fourth arm to retract and counter-retract the breast parenchyma (Fig. 9-8).

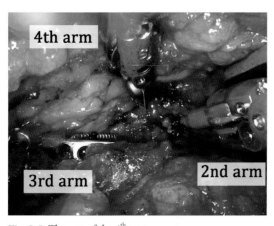

Fig. 9-8. The use of the 4th arm

Console

Using the robotic arms, the superficial subcutaneous flap is dissected below the nipple-areolar complex to the breast borders, including the outer, inner, upper, and lower margins. An assistant checks the state of the flap by observing the degree of illumination (visual inspection). If the retromammary space is not fully dissected before docking, the deep layer of the superficial fascia in the retromammary space is subsequently dissected from the lateral margin of the pectoral muscle fascia to the entire deep layer of the retromammary tissues. When full mobilization of the breast parenchyma is completed, the specimen can be easily removed through the axillary incision.

Specimen retrieval

After robot docking is released, the specimen is retrieved through the incision.

After the retrieval of the specimen

The surgical margins of the specimen are inspected and palpated. If you suspect the surgical margins may have tumor involvement, intraoperative frozen section of the surgical margin can be helpful to identify tumor involvement. This is similar with the gas technique. After the completion of the mastectomy, immediate reconstruction begins.

REFERENCES

1. Randall P, Dabb R, Loc N. "Apple coring" the nipple in subcutaneous mastectomy. Plastic and reconstructive surgery. 1979;64(6):800-3.

10. Gasless Endoscopy-Assisted Nipple-Sparing Mastectomy

Hyung Seok Park

Position, Incision design, Marking of borders, and Sentinel lymph node biopsy

The position, incision design, marking of borders, and sentinel lymph node biopsy are performed in the same manner as the gasless robot-assisted Nipple-Sparing mastectomy. An incision of at least 6 cm at the anterior axillary line is recommended for the gasless endoscopic nipple-sparing mastectomy. For a beginner, the position of the incision of the gasless endoscopic nipple-sparing mastectomy can be located at a location 1-2 cm more anterior to the anterior axillary line than the gas-inflated or gasless robot nipple-sparing mastectomy. Because endoscopic mastectomy uses rigid endoscopic devices which have fewer degrees of freedom in the instruments than robotic surgical systems, a longer and more anteriorly located incision is recommended for easier approach using endoscopic devices.

Subcutaneous flap and retromammary space dissection

After the sentinel lymph node biopsy, subcutaneous flap dissection toward the nipple-areolar complex is prepared through the incision using an electrocautery and/or an advanced energy device, such as ultrasonic vessel shears or bipolar vessel sealing devices. Using advanced energy devices can make it easier to dissect the subcutaneous flap and retromammary space. Undermining of a subcutaneous flap to the nipple-areolar complex from the axilla can be performed through a sharp dissection using a monopolar electrocautery. The subcutaneous flap should be performed as much as possible to be able to insert the self-refractor called 'Chung's retractor' (Fig. 9-7). The remaining subcutaneous flap, which is difficult to dissect through manual sharp dissection using monopolar electrocautery, can be bluntly dissected using Metzenbaum scissors after tumescent solution injection. The whole subcutaneous flap can be dissected by either sharp or blunt dissection. Bleeding in the superficial flap can be controlled by monopolar electrocautery or advanced energy devices.

Dissection of nipple-areolar complex

Nipple-areolar complex can be dissected through the 6 cm axillary incision. This procedure is performed similarly to the gasless robotic nipple-sparing mastectomy.

Application of a self-retractor

A self-retractor is inserted below the subcutaneous flap. If you appropriately dissected the whole superficial flap and retromammary space before the application of the self-retractor, the remaining tissue of the breast parenchyma will be in the upper, inner, and lower parts of the breast (Fig. 10-1). The remaining tissue can be dissected by endoscopy, endoscopic forceps, endoscopic monopolar curved scissors, and/or an advanced energy device with a long shaft. Advanced energy devices with long shafts are useful to dissect the deep inner area of the breast parenchyma (Fig. 10-2).

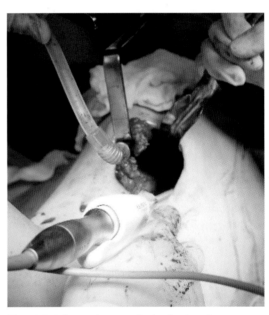

Fig. 10-2. Advanced energy device for deep inner area

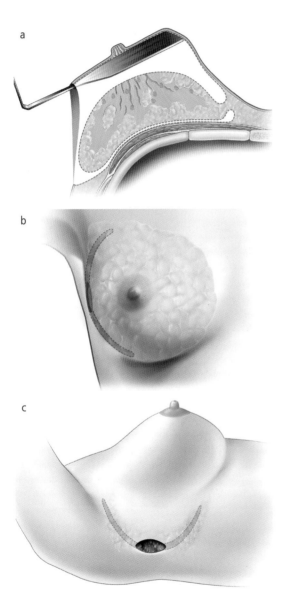

Fig. 10-1. Superficial flap dissection
a. Transverse view
b. Anterior view
c. Lateral view

Specimen retrieval

The specimen is retrieved through the incision. Procedures after the retrieval of the specimen are similar with those of the RNSM (After the retrieval of the specimen, chapter 8. p.86).

11. Robot-Assisted Nipple-Sparing Mastectomy Using the Single Port System

Hyung Seok Park

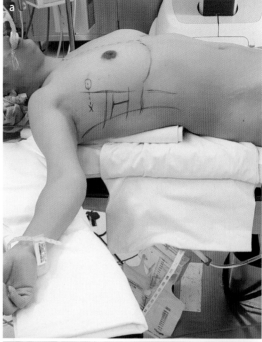

Position

The patient's position in the RNSM using the SP system is different from that in the RNSM using the multiport systems including Xi and Si. Because the patient cart of the SP system has a single cannula, collisions between robotic arms, which can occur in the RNSM using multiport systems, do not occur in the SP system. The patient is placed in the supine position with 90–100 degree arm abduction over an arm-board (Fig. 11-1).

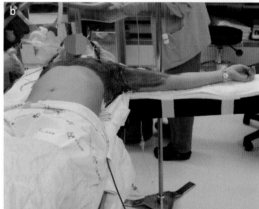

A shoulder pad or pillow can be inserted under the back of the patient to slightly elevate the upper trunk. It is unnecessary to mount a raised arm board (Mizuho Medical Co., Tokyo, Japan) because collisions between robot and patient arms also rarely occur when the position is appropriate. A guiding principle when positioning the instrument drive is to secure enough space between the instrument drive and patient arm over the arm-board.

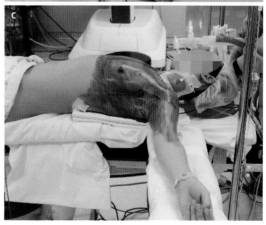

Fig. 11-1. Positioning for SP system

Incision design

The actual incision line is drawn using a marker pen. The incision should be no more than 3 cm to avoid air leakage. The optimal incision for RNSM using the SP system is 2.5–3.5 cm. If additional incision length is required for the axillary lymph node dissection, additional sutures around the single port device are necessary to prevent air leakage. Otherwise, you can extend the incision length when you retrieve the specimen. You can also perform axillary lymph node dissection through the extended incision after the retrieval of the specimen. The length of the extended incision depends on breast volume/weight(Table 8-1).

Marking of borders

Breast borders are lined using a marker pen (Fig. 8-10). For sentinel lymph node biopsy and border-marking, blue dye is injected into the periareolar area and breast borders. (Fig. 8-11). A 28G short needle and syringe should be used for blue dye injection into the borders because a larger and longer needle can cause iatrogenic pneumothorax (Fig. 8-12, 13). Blue dye injection for the breast border-marking is made into at least twelve points around the borders with 2–3 cm distance between each injection (Fig. 8-12, 14).

Sentinel lymph node biopsy

After the incision is made, sentinel lymph node biopsy is performed. Senn or small Richardson retractors are applied to approach the axilla (Fig. 8-15). When the clavicopectoral fascia is identified, a gamma probe is applied to detect sentinel lymph nodes (Fig. 8-16). Because of the longer distance between the incision and the axillary area than in conventional sentinel lymph node biopsy, advanced energy devices including HARMONIC ACE® +7 Shears with Advanced Hemostasis (Ethicon Inc., Cornelia, GA, USA) and Ligasure™ Maryland Jaw Device with Nano-Coated Jaws (Medtronic, Minneapolis, MN, USA) can be used (Fig. 8-17, 18). Advanced energy devices enable easier dissection and hemostasis for sentinel lymph node biopsy. Fiberoptic retractors can be used for better visualization of the operation field during sentinel lymph node biopsy (Fig. 8-19, 20). Intraoperative frozen section can be used to identify the involvement of metastatic cells in the sentinel lymph nodes. If metastasis is identified in a sentinel lymph node, conventional or robotic axillary lymph node dissection can be performed through the extended incision.

Creation of working space and retromammary space dissection

After the sentinel lymph node biopsy, the working space should be made (Fig. 8-22~25). The estimated area of the working space is marked with the wound protector using a marker pen (Fig. 8-23). Working space is created by manual dissection using a monopolar electrocautery. Both the superficial layer and retromammary space are manually dissected as much as possible.

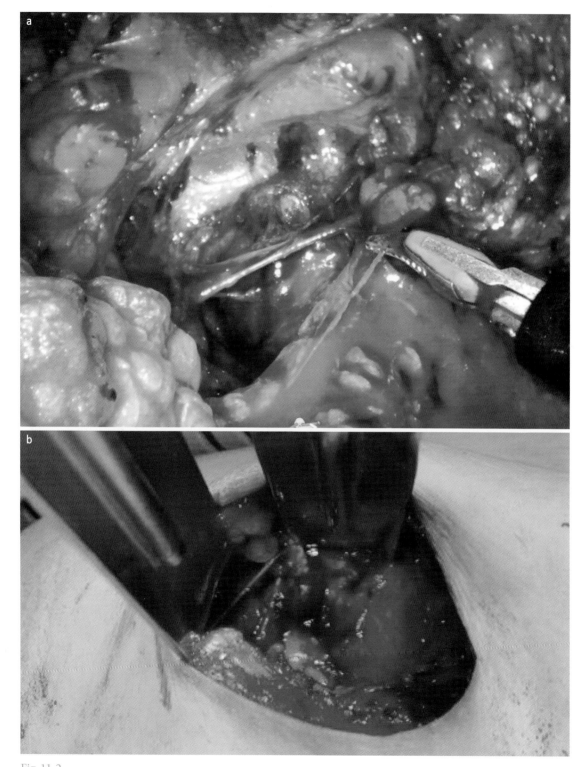

Fig. 11-2.
a. View of robotic axillary lymph node dissection
b. Conventional axillary lymph node dissection through the incision for RNSM

Injection of the tumescent solution

The tumescent solution is injected into the superficial layer of the superficial fascia. Tunneling under the subcutaneous tissue is performed using Metzenbaum scissors (Fig. 8-32). After tunneling, the remaining tumescent solution is pushed out to the incision site by rolling gauze or a sponge along the breast (Fig. 8-33).

Attachment of single port device

An Alexis® O wound protector or UNI-PORT wound retractor is placed in the working space. A cannula of the robotic system is inserted to the GelPoint® or UNI-PORT that is attached to the wound protector. The patient cart is placed at the opposite side of the operation field (Fig. 8-37). An additional 5 mm port is inserted into the GelPoint or UNI-PORT beside the cannula of the robotic system.

Hanging suture for pulling of nipple-areolar complex

Hanging suture is performed to pull up the nipple-areolar complex to avoid injury during robotic dissection of the subareolar tissue (Fig. 8-36).

Docking

A camera is installed in the camera port. da Vinci SP® fenestrated bipolar forceps (FBF), da Vinci SP® Maryland bipolar forceps (MBF) or Cardiere, and Da Vinci SP® monopolar curved scissors (MCS) are mounted on arms 1, 2, and 3, respectively.

Console

The robotic arms are controlled by the operator on the console. The subcutaneous flap is dissected using MCS with counter-retraction using FBF. The camera can stand in the cobra position for the dissection of the medial area (Fig. 11-3)

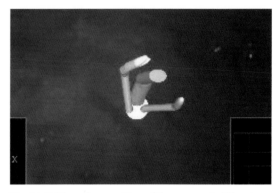

Fig. 11-3. The cobra position of the camera in SP system

When the blue dye is identified along the medial border, the dissection should be stopped. The upper and lower subcutaneous flap dissections are performed in a similar manner. After the completion of the subcutaneous flap dissections, instrument drives are rotated 180°, and the camera drive is placed in the lower position. The remaining retromammary tissue is dissected using MCS, with counter-retraction using FBF and Maryland forceps.

Specimen retrieval

After full detachment of the breast parenchyma, the robotic docking is released to obtain the specimen. Usually, the 2.5-3.0

cm incision size is too small to retrieve the specimen. The initial incision can be extended to retrieve the specimen. The length of incision extension depends on the breast volume/weight of the patient.

After the retrieval of the specimen

Inspection or palpation of the surgical margins of the breast tissue helps confirm grossly safe margins. Frozen section for the surgical margins can be applied if a lesion is suspected. Additional subcutaneous flap dissection can be manually performed using Metzenbaum scissors or an electrocautery to achieve oncologic safety when the subcutaneous flap is thicker than 5 mm or when there is tumor involvement in the superficial margins.

The pocket of the prepectoral space can be irrigated using normal saline. Inspection with fiberoptic retractors into the pocket of the prepectoral space is important for finding hidden bleeding sites. When mastectomy is completed, immediate breast reconstruction begins.

Immediate Prosthetic Breast Reconstruction

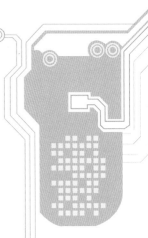

12. Introduction of Prosthetic Breast Reconstruction

Seung Yong Song

Prosthetic reconstruction is the most commonly conducted breast reconstruction method in most countries. In prosthetic reconstruction, tissue expanders or breast implants, which are usually made with silicone, are commonly used to reconstruct the removed breast.

This method is more simple than autologous free flap methods. Autologous free flap techniques need special surgical instruments or techniques, such as dopplers, microscopes and microsurgical techniques, which require additional training and have learning curves. Meanwhile, for prosthetic reconstruction, special surgical instruments or techniques are unnecessary, so surgeons can relatively easily perform this type of reconstruction. Nevertheless, abundant experience and knowledge is also necessary to improve patient safety and satisfaction.

Prosthetic reconstruction has other advantages including short operation time, smaller scars and shorter recovery time. Disadvantages of this technique include the risk of infection, capsular contracture, and anaplastic large cell lymphoma in specific types of implant.

Classification

Prosthetic breast reconstruction can be classified into one-stage and two-stage reconstructions. In two-stage reconstructions, a tissue expander is inserted into sub- or pre-pectoral pockets at the first stage operation, and after expanding the overlying skin, the tissue expander is removed and permanent implant is inserted in the pockets at the second stage operation. Two-stage subpectoral breast reconstruction is considered to be the standard method of prosthetic breast reconstruction because of its safety.[1-3]

In contrast, in one-stage breast reconstruction, the permanent implant is directly inserted into the appropriate pocket without tissue expansion. This method is enabled by the increased use of Nipple-Sparing mastectomy and acellular dermal matrix.[4] This method is also called direct-to-implant (DTI) procedure.

Determination of prosthetic breast reconstruction method after robot-assisted nipple-sparing mastectomy

After RNSM, both one or two-stage options are available. Generally, there is a consensus that two-stage prosthetic reconstruction tends to have a higher rate of satisfaction from paitents and fewer complications.[3] In particular, mastectomy flap ischemia and necrosis can be minimized by two-stage procedures. However, if surgeons can appropriately select patients with less risk of flap ischemia and necrosis, DTI can provide comparable results to two-stage breast reconstruction (Fig. 12-1).[5] Fortunately, we have found that DTI procedure with appropriate patient selection has a relatively low risk of nipple necrosis in our experience.

Evaluation of vascular perfusion of mastectomy flap

To identify the amount of vascular perfusion to the whole mastectomy flap including skin and nipple-areolar complex, we recommend using indocyanine green (ICG) video angiography before deciding the reconstruction method. This device is

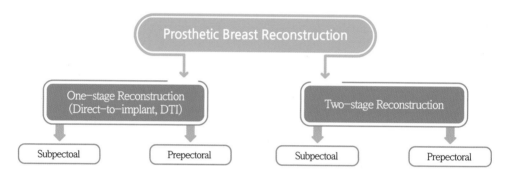

Fig. 12-1. Schematic diagram of prosthetic breast reconstruction option after robot-assisted mastectomy

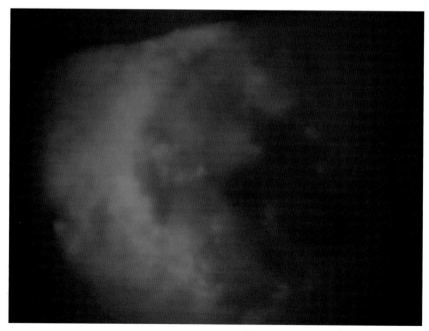

Fig. 12-2. ICG video angiography using FLUOBEAM in Lt. robot-assisted mastectomy case, Rt. black area indicates vascular insufficiency.

commonly used to determine flap perfusion area or lymphatic flow.[6] It is also useful to determine nipple viability or mastectomy flap perfusion after RNSM.

If perfusion to skin and the nipple area is confirmed, DTI can be performed with relatively low complication risk. If there is a wide area of non-perfusion detected around the nipple, tissue expander insertion for two-stage reconstruction should be considered rather than DTI (Fig. 12-2).

Robot prosthetic breast reconstruction

Robotic surgical systems can be used in prosthetic reconstruction. Specifically, pectoralis major dissection, acellular dermal matrix (ADM) fixation, and inframammary fold (IMF) fixation can be performed using robotic surgical systems. All of these procedures can be done manually with long instruments in some cases by experienced surgeons; however, in other cases, it is not feasible or even possible in some cases because surgical views are limited due to small incisions and chest wall curvatures. These limitations lead to incomplete dissection, malposition of ADM, and difficulties in identification and coagulation of intercostal perforator vessels.

The author has experience with da Vinci Si, Xi, and daVinci SP (Intuitive Surgical Inc. Sunnyvale, CA). Da Vinci SP is more suitable for breast surgeries because it allows dissection and fixation in limited spaces and via small incisions.

REFERENCES

1. McCarthy CM, Mehrara BJ, Riedel E, Davidge K, Hinson A, Disa JJ, et al. Predicting complications following expander/implant breast reconstruction: an outcomes analysis based on preoperative clinical risk. Plastic and reconstructive surgery. 2008;121(6):1886-92.

2. Ahn SJ, Woo TY, Lee DW, Lew DH, Song SY. Nipple-areolar complex ischemia and necrosis in nipple-sparing mastectomy. European journal of surgical oncology : the journal of the European Society of Surgical Oncology and the British Association of Surgical Oncology. 2018;44(8):1170-6.

3. Negenborn VL, Young Afat DA, Dikmans REG, Smit JM, Winters HAH, Don Griot JPW, et al. Quality of life and patient satisfaction after one-stage implant-based breast reconstruction with an acellular dermal matrix versus two-stage breast reconstruction (BRIOS): primary outcome of a randomised, controlled trial. Lancet oncology. 2018;19(9):1205-14.

4. Salzberg CA, Ashikari AY, Koch RM, Chabner Thompson E. An 8-year experience of direct-to-implant immediate breast reconstruction using human acellular dermal matrix (AlloDerm). Plastic & Reconstructive Surgery. 2011;127(2):514-24.

5. Srinivasa DR, Garvey PB, Qi J, Hamill JB, Kim HM, Pusic AL, et al. Direct-to-Implant versus Two-Stage Tissue Expander/Implant Reconstruction: 2-Year Risks and Patient-Reported Outcomes from a Prospective, Multicenter Study. Plastic & Reconstructive Surgery. 2017;140(5):869-77.

6. Lee SK, Lee DW, Lew DH, Song SY. Determining the Trimming Layer in Breast Reconstruction with a Free TRAM Flap Using Intraoperative Video-angiography. Plastic and Reconstructive Surgery-Global Open. 2017;5(3):e1266-e.

13. Two-stage breast Reconstruction

Seung Yong Song and Hyung Seok Park

Since the first introduction of two-stage breast reconstruction by C. Radovan in 1982, this method has been considered to be the standard option by many reconstructive surgeons. Radovan used the subpectoral pocket for implant placement. However, due to the development of acellular dermal matrix (ADM), prepectoral pocket implant is also a viable option.[1, 2]

In fact, RNSM preserves the nipple-areolar complex, and hence, the necessity of two-stage breast reconstruction has decreased. However, two-stage reconstruction is still performed for some patients.

In general, we prefer one-stage reconstruction because of surgical difficulties in the second stage operation. Second stage operation for permanent implant insertion often requires additional procedures, including capsulectomy, capsulotomy, capsulorraphy, and/or inframammary fold repositioning. The small laterally located incision of RNSM makes these procedures more difficult. These difficulties can be directly associated with various surgical complications and less patient satisfaction.

Therefore, we recommend DTI after robot-assisted mastectomy whenever possible. Two-stage breast reconstruction should be conducted in some particular situations, such as situations where patients want contralateral breast augmentation or where mastectomy flap perfusion is markedly decreased.

Subpectoral two-stage reconstruction
First stage for tissue expander insertion

The author (SYS) prefers to use ADM for lower pole coverage. Pectoralis major muscle elevation and ADM fixation can be conducted either by robotic surgical systems or manually. It is challenging to perform these procedures manually when the incision is located more laterally or is smaller. One of the main problems of tissue expander insertion using robotic surgical systems is that it is difficult for surgeons to identify the exact location within the breast pocket. Skin or soft tissue marking with temporary vital blue dye, such as indigo carmine, and help from an assistant next to the patient can be helpful to reduce the difficulty (Fig. 13-1).

The incision may need to be extended due to the presence of the injection port of the tissue expander.

Second stage for tissue expander removal and permanent implant insertion

The second stage operation is somewhat challenging because of visual limitations and small working space for surgical devices due to the laterally located small incision.

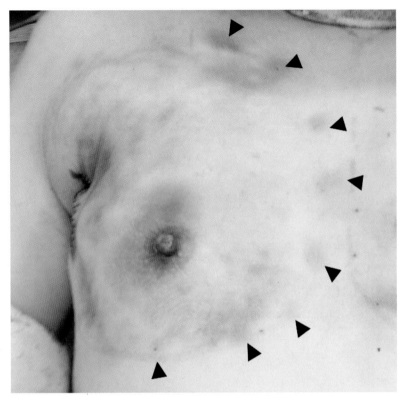

Fig. 13-1. Surgical margins were marked with indigocarmine (skyblue stained spots pointed by black arrows) Indigocarmine is injected into not only skin but subcutaneous fat and/or muscle. These markings can guide both oncologic surgeons and reconstructive surgeons.

In this stage, robotic systems have not been used because capsule work and positioning of implant usually require multiple patient position changes for operative accuracy. In the author's (SYS) opinion, robot docking and removal are cumbersome processes, so using robotic systems in the second stage operation may not be appropriate.

The second procedure can be conducted manually. It requires long shaft instruments like monopolar coagulator, needle holder, and forceps. In most cases, manual capsulectomy, capsulotomy, capsulorraphy, and inframammary fold repositioning after

RNSM can be done with longer instruments following the surgeon's preference. However, they require longer operation time compared to second-stage operation after conventional nipple-sparing mastectomy.

Unfortunately, the surgeon cannot have a comfortable position during the manual prodecure due to the narrow working space. Hence, it will get challenging if the surgeon needs to perform revision surgeries due to complications, such as capsular contracture or animation deformity of the second-stage operation. Endoscopic devices can facilitate these surgical procedures (Fig. 13-2). However,

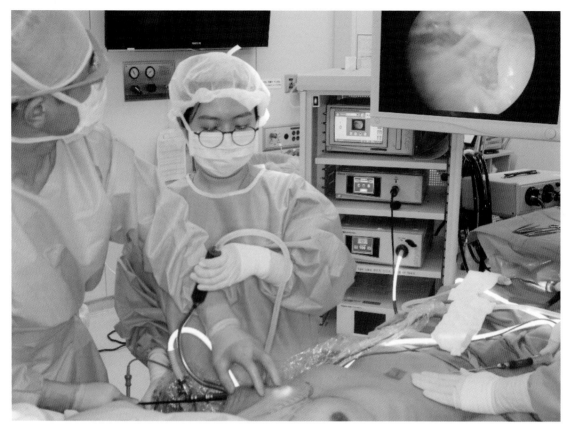

Fig. 13-2. Second stage operation for tissue expander removal and permanent implant insertion using endoscope.

there is a learning curve for endoscopic surgery, and this should be performed with caution not to perforate the breast skin envelope.

For these reasons, subpectoral pocket for implant insertion may not be the most ideal option after robot-assisted mastectomies.

Additional procedures including fat graft are also possible at this stage.

Prepectoral two-stage reconstruction
First stage for tissue expander insertion

Prepectoral tissue expander insertion is more similar to DTI rather than subpectoral tissue expander insertion. Due to the small incision, the collapsed nature of the tissue expander, and the risk of expander injury during ADM fixation, it is difficult to apply the 'anterior coverage technique' for tissue expander insertion (Fig. 13-3). In contrast, the ADM wrapping technique is viable for tissue expander insertion after robot-assisted mastectomy (Fig. 13-4). However, it is not easy to cover a tissue expander with ADM and to insert the ADM-wrapped tissue expander into the prepectoral pocket through a small incision. To insert the wrapped expander, an incision of at least 4-5cm is needed. Surgeons

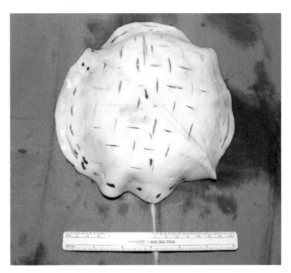

Fig. 13-3. Anterior coverage technique

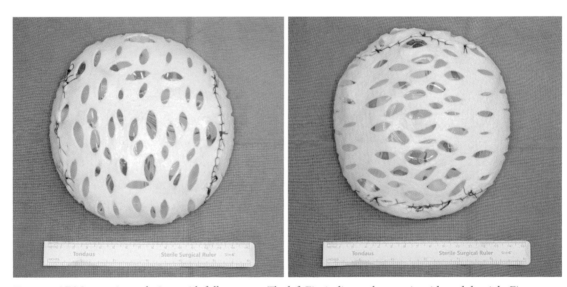

Fig. 13-4. ADM wrapping technique with full coverage. The left Fig. indicates the anterior side and the right Fig. indicates posterior side of the implant with ADM

should be careful to locate the tissue expander at the proper position and not to rupture the ADM during fixation sutures.

To insert the tissue expander prepectorally, the author (SYS) prefers to fill the expander with normal saline until near full expansion because the ADM should be fitted to the fully inflated expander. The ADM is wrapped around the expander and fixed with absorbable sutures. After the expander is wrapped, it is deflated again to be inserted into the pocket through the small incision. After irrigating the pocket, two drains are placed: one is located in the inframammary fold and the other is located in the axilla and cephalic margin of the expander. The expander is inserted into the pocket using a hyaluronic acid-coated funnel to facilitate this process.

Second stage for tissue expander removal and permanent implant insertion

In prepectoral implant insertion, ADM work is important for proper implant positioning and lower pole expansion. In this regard, it is not easy to do these ADM manipulations through a laterally located short incision, as opposed to ADM manipulations after conventional NSM. More caution should be given not to perforate the skin flap because only a thin layer of skin remains outside of the ADM in contrast to the subpectoral procedure. In many cases, the pocket that is made by ADM does not exactly match with the desired permanent implant pocket. Therefore, some portion of the ADM should be incised, removed, or reduced. These procedures are also challenging because of the laterally located short incision. Endoscopy can facilitate these procedures if the surgeon is skillful at manipulating endoscopic devices. These surgical procedures like ADM manipulations and pocket control can be performed manually using longer surgical devices with careful skills.

Advantages and preferred patient selection of two-stage breast reconstruction

Because there is less skin tension in two-stage reconstruction compared to one-stage reconstruction, improved nipple or mastectomy flap viability can be expected.[3] Modification of the implant pocket for proper implant positioning is possible at the second stage operation. More precise and symmetric implant selection can be achieved based on the previous expander position and volume in the second stage operation.

The author (SYS) prefers to perform two-stage breast reconstruction in some selected situations. Patients with insufficient vascular perfusion of the skin after RNSM are candidates for two-stage breast reconstruction. The vascular insufficiency can be determined by ICG video angiography or discussion with the breast oncologic surgeons regarding the intraoperative findings. However, possibility of inserting a tissue expander instead of a permanent implant should be informed to the patients before the definitive surgery. Patients who want contralateral breast augmentation in the second stage operation are also preferred candidates for this procedure.

Step-by-step procedures for tissue expander insertion

Robot-assisted subpectoral tissue expander insertion

(1) Confirmation of vascular perfusion with ICG video angiography

(2) Patient position

For the insertion of the tissue expander, there is no need to change the patient's position that was set by oncologic surgeons for mastectomy. The arm at the operative side is fully abducted and fixed, and the patient's body is tilted slightly to the non-operative side.

(3) Preparation of operative field

Gas and gasless retraction are both possible. We prefer the preparation of CO_2 gas inflation to gain a proper operative field. The incision is covered with the UNI-PORT (Dalim Medical Corporation, Gyeonggi-do, Korea). The author (SYS) usually prefers to set the pressure of CO_2 gas at 8 mmHg. The range of the pressure is 8–12 mmHg.

(4) Pectoralis muscle flap elevation

Manual dissection is possible in the beginning. When we think of the mastectomized space as a clock, the area from 6 to 12 o'clock of the right breast can be dissected manually. However, the area from 12 to 6 o'clock needs robotic dissection due to chest wall curvature and the long distance from the entrance. (inside of the yellow line in Fig. 13-5) For the dissection of this area, the author (SYS) prefers

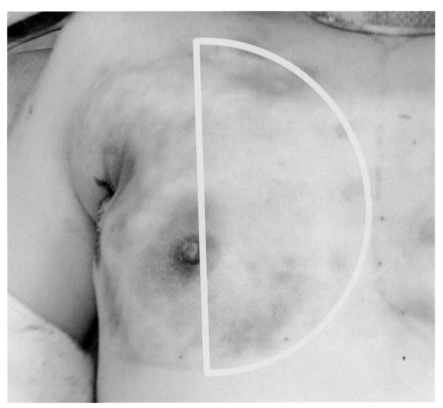

Fig. 13-5. Inside of the yellow line indicates the area which needs robotic dissection (12-6 o'clock). The remaining half (6 to 12 o'clock) can be accessed manually.

to use fenestrated bipolar forceps (Intuitive Surgical Inc., Sunnyvale, CA) with the non-dominant hand and Maryland bipolar forceps (Intuitive Surgical Inc., Sunnyvale, CA) with the dominant hand. To ligate large vessels, bipolar coagulation by the robotic surgical system can be used. Surgical clips can be helpful as well. Erbe bipolar coagulator (Erbe Elektromedizin GmbH, Tuebingen, Germany) is to be set to power four.

(5) Lower pole coverage with ADM

After dissection, ADM can be introduced into the lower pole of the breast. Prograsp forceps (Intuitive Surgical Inc., Sunnyvale, CA) are used with the non-dominant hand and large needle drivers (Intuitive Surgical Inc., Sunnyvale, CA) are used with the dominant hand for ADM fixation. The fixation point can be indicated with indigo carmine or the assistant's finger outside of the pocket. About three points of the medial margin of the breast (3 to 6 o'clock) are fixed by sutures using the robotic surgical system. Additional fixations near the operator's side can be performed manually. Sutures between the pectoralis major and the lateral portion of ADM are not fixed before the introduction of the tissue expander because the pocket opening is essential for insertion of the folded expander and prevention of ruptures of fixation sutures.

(6) Introduction of tissue expander

Tissue expander can be inserted after deflation and folding. A hyaluronic acid-coated funnel can facilitate this process. After insertion of the tissue expander, the lateral margin of the ADM can be fixed to the pectoralis major muscle. Then, the pectoralis major and ADM are approximated with absorbable sutures. Be cautious during these procedures because the expander can be easily ruptured by the suture needles. Using a spatula can be helpful to effectively protect the expander.

When fixing large expanders in large breast pockets, medial sutures between the pectoralis major and the ADM are difficult to perform. In this case, some stitches between the pectoralis major and the ADM before gently inserting the tissue expander into the pocket can be helpful.

(7) Placement of drains

The author (SYS) prefers inserting two drains which are placed in the inframammary fold and the axilla to the anterior area of the pectoralis muscle, respectively.

(8) Skin repair

Usually, the soft and subcutaneous tissues near the latissimus dorsi muscle that are located posteriorly to the incision move posteriorly due to the gravity in the supine position. Therefore, proper fixation of the posterior tissue near the incision site is important in achieving good patient satisfaction. Skin is approximated with nylon sutures or skin adhesives.

Manual subpectoral tissue expander insertion

Generally, all procedures are the same with the insertion of tissue expander using robotic surgical systems. For the manual insertion of tissue expanders, long surgical instruments such as DeBakey forceps or long needle holders are useful.

The author (SYS) thinks that it is difficult to perform this procedure manually. However, all procedures can be performed without the assistance of robotic surgical systems. If the incision is too small to perform the insertion of the tissue expander manually, you can extend the incision made by the oncologic surgeon in RNSM by 1-2 cm.

Second stage operation for tissue expander removal and permanent implant insertion

(1) Patient position

The position of the patient is the same as that in the first stage operation. The arm at the operative side is fully abducted and fixed. The patient's body is tilted to the non-operative side.

(2) Removal of tissue expander

The previous incision is reopened. The border of ADM and the serratus muscle is incised and the capsule is opened. The expander is deflated with negative pressure suction. After complete deflation, the expander is folded in the pocket and removed by pulling with a gentle external pressure.

(3) Pocket control

Necessary capsule work can be performed with long forceps and an electrocautery or with the assistance of endoscopic devices. Special attention should be paid not to perforate the envelope especially in the medial area of the breasts.

(4) Placement of drain

The author (SYS) prefers one drain with sufficient length at the inframammary fold.

(5) Introduction of permanent implant

An implant of an appropriate size can be introduced into the pocket. To prevent implant fracture and possible contamination from the normal flora of the skin, we recommend the use of a hyaluronic acid-coated funnel.

(6) Closure of skin

If subcutaneous tissue near the incision site moves from its original position, fixation with subcutaneous tissue helps prevent skin depression around the implant. If the incision margin is macerated due to extensive retracting, revision will be necessary to facilitate wound healing.

(7) Postoperative care

Avoid excessive pressure because the thin skin flap can be necrotized by ischemia. The drain is usually removed when the daily amount of drainage is less than 30cc with a clear decreasing trend of drainage volumes.

REFERENCES

1. Radovan C. Breast reconstruction after mastectomy using the temporary expander. Plastic & Reconstructive Surgery. 1982;69(2):195-208.

2. Sbitany H, Piper M, Lentz R. Prepectoral Breast Reconstruction: A Safe Alternative to Submuscular Prosthetic Reconstruction following Nipple-Sparing Mastectomy. Plastic & Reconstructive Surgery. 2017;140(3):432-43.

3. Yang C, Chung SW, Lee DW, Lew DH, Song SY. Evaluation of the Relationship Between Flap Tension and Tissue Perfusion in Implant-Based Breast Reconstruction Using Laser-Assisted Indocyanine Green Angiography. Annals of Surgical Oncology. 2018;25(8):2235-40.

14. One-stage Breast Reconstruction, Direct-to-Implant

Seung Yong Song and Hyung Seok Park

Direct-to-implant (DTI) reconstruction can reduce surgery times and hospital visits. DTI reconstruction shows favorable patient satisfaction compared to two-stage breast reconstruction when the patient is appropriately selected.[1, 2]

One-stage breast reconstruction without ADM was introduced at the early period of breast reconstruction. This method was associated with high rates of complications including exposure, capsular contracture, malposition, and rippling. In contrast, the two-stage subpectoral implantation with an additional subserratus pocket showed low rates of complications. Therefore, two-stage reconstruction has been considered as the standard method for several decades.[3]

However, one-stage reconstruction has recently been brought back into focus with the advent of acellular dermal matrix (ADM) and the increased rate of Nipple-Sparing mastectomy. One-stage reconstruction is becoming more popular with reconstructive surgeons because it reduces the patient's burden of additional anesthesia and economic and social costs of tissue expansion.

DTI was first achieved using the subpectoral technique. The origin of the pectoralis major muscle is detached and the lateral and caudal area of the implant is covered by the ADM sling. This method yields acceptable results not inferior to two-stage reconstruction in aspects of complication rates and patient satisfaction.[4]

Prepectoral DTI was also introduced after the application of the DTI with the subpectoral technique. There are two ADM wrapping methods for implant in the prepectoral DTI technique. Some surgeons prefer fully wrapped implants and some prefer partial anterior-wrapped implants.[5, 6]

Most robot-assisted mastectomies are Nipple-Sparing mastectomies. RNSM has a high possibility of nipple survival because there is no incision around the nipple. Moreover, due to difficulties in surgical procedures via the small incision of RNSM in second stage operation, we believe that DTI is the most suitable option for breast prosthetic reconstruction after RNSM.

Subpectoral DTI

The subpectoral placement of a permanent implant is a viable option after RNSM. Surgical procedures are largely similar to the subpectoral insertion of tissue expanders, but more accurate implant selection and manipulation of the implant pocket dissection are necessary.

Pectoralis muscle dissection and ADM

fixation are conducted with robot-assistance. In the authors' experience, manual dissection and ADM fixation were possible in more than half of the cases. However, it was difficult because of the small incision, curvature of the anterior chest wall, and long distance of the surgical field from the incision.

Prepectoral DTI

The author (SYS) considers the prepectoral insertion of ADM-wrapped permanent implant to be the best method of prosthetic reconstruction after RNSM. The reason is that the preprectoal DTI technique is not only easy and fast, but also not inferior to the other methods in terms of complication rates. Furthermore, it provides high patient satisfaction.

Intraoperatively, secure fixation of the ADM is essential because stitches can rupture during the introduction of the wrapped implant into the pocket via the small incision. A hyaluronic acid-coated funnel can reduce these difficulties.

After RNSM, patients usually have a larger pocket than the implant dimensions. Therefore, implants can migrate into unwanted space and malposition can occur.

In contrast, although mastectomy flap perfusion after robot-assisted mastectomy is usually good, there can be more injured tissues suffering from arterial and venous insufficiency compared to normal breasts. Direct pressure from the elastic compressive bandage application, which usually is not considered to be heavy or harmful under normal conditions, may damage the thin mastectomy flap. The direct pressure to the flap might be associated with complications including nipple and skin necrosis which can cause failure of the reconstruction. This is a potential concern of the prepectoral prosthetic reconstruction after RNSM.

To achieve low complication rates and aesthetically pleasing results, the author (SYS) focuses on improving the survival the mastectomy flap for 3-5 days postoperatively.

If there is no problem in the flap perfusion, more active measures like the elastic compressive bandage are applied for maintaining the proper pocket formation.

The author (SYS) prefers to use nitric oxide (NO) ointments and hyperbaric oxygen therapy if the nipple viability looks compromised. If there is a serious situation of ischemic change of the skin and nipple in the early post-operative period, changing from implant to tissue expander under general anesthesia can be considered. If there is no serious event of ischemia of the skin and nipple, a tighter brassiere with an upper bandage can be worn.

Advantages of DTI

DTI is one of the ideal breast reconstruction methods because patients can have reduced operation time and hospital stay. DTI minimizes the psychological stress of mastectomy and reconstruction.[2, 4]

However, in cases of prepectoral DTI,

the cost of ADM is high, which can be an economic barrier for this technique.

Indications of DTI
- Sufficient vascular perfusion of mastectomized flap: patients with good perfusion in ICG video angiography.
- Patients who do not require contralateral balancing procedures.
- Small to medium size breasts. However, large breasts can be candidates if perfusion is good.

Step-by-Step Procedures for DTI
Robot-assisted subpectoral permanent implant insertion

(1) Confirmation of vascular perfusion with ICG video angiography

(2) Fixation of the inframammary fold

In this step, the surgeon should confirm whether the inframammary fold (IMF) is intact. To investigate the integrity of the IMF, the author (SYS) recommends inserting breast implant sizers into the pocket. By inserting sizers, the destruction of the IMF is easily identified, and it can also help in selection of an implant of proper dimension and volume.

New fixation of IMF requires effort and time; therefore, it is most desirable that IMF is not destroyed during oncologic surgery. However, there is always a possibility of these events because oncologic surgeons cannot see the outside of the breasts during robotic surgery. Therefore, markings with indigo carmine or the assistance of the 1st assistant

are necessary to preserve the IMF.

If IMF has been destroyed, proper position of IMF by fixation using absorbable sutures is essential to achieve breast symmetry and cosmesis. This process can be performed using robotic surgical systems or manual fixation using long forceps and needle holders. In subpectoral DTI, IMF can be determined by fixation of the caudal edge of ADM and the chest wall or the anterior breast envelope and the chest wall.

(3) Patient position

The patient's position for the subpectoral DTI reconstruction is the same as that for the tissue expander insertion. The oncologic surgeon's setting of the patient's position is suitable for the subpectoral DTI insertion.

(4) Preparation of the operative field

Gas and gasless are both possible. We prefer the preparation of CO_2 gas inflation to gain a proper operative field. The incision is covered with the UNI-PORT. The author (SYS) usually prefers to set the pressure of CO_2 gas at 8mmHg. The range of the pressure is 8–12 mmHg (Same with chapter 13, page 112.).

(5) Pectoralis muscle flap elevation

Manual dissection is possible at the beginning of the procedure. The area making up the 6 to 12 o'clock of the right breast can be dissected manually. However, the medial area of the right breast, from 12 to 6 o'clock area, needs robotic dissection due to the chest wall curvature and long distance from the entrance. Instrument setting is the same with previous description chapter 13, page 112.

(6) Lower pole coverage with ADM

After dissection, ADM can be introduced into the lower pole of the breast. Prograsp forceps (Intuitive Surgical Inc., Sunnyvale, CA) in the non-dominant hand and large needle drivers (Intuitive Surgical Inc., Sunnyvale, CA) in the dominant hand is the preferable setting for ADM fixation. The fixation point can be guided with injected blue dye or by the assistant's finger outside of the pocket. About three points of the lower medial border of the breast (3 to 6 o'clock of the right breast) are sutured using robotic surgical systems. The remaining fixation can be performed manually. Sutures between the pectoralis major and lateral portion of ADM are described in the chapter 13, page 113.

(7) Introduction of permanent implant

A hyaluronic acid-coated funnel can facilitate this process. After the insertion of the implant, the lateral margin of ADM can be fixed and then the pectoralis major and ADM can be approximated with absorbable sutures. Caution should be made during this procedure not to rupture the implant. Spatulas can effectively protect implants from rupturing.

(8) Placement of drains

The author (SYS) prefers two drains, one for the inframammary fold, the other for the axilla and anterior area of the pectoralis muscle.

(9) Skin repair

Skin repair is performed in the same manner as other prosthetic reconstructions after RNSM chapter 13, page 113-114.

Manual subpectoral permanent implant insertion

Generally, all procedures are the same with robot-assisted implant insertion. In this manual method, longer surgical instruments are useful.

(1) Prepectoral ADM-wrapped permanent implant insertion without robot
  i) Evaluation of vascular perfusion using ICG video angiography
  ii) Fixation of the inframammary fold
    The fixation of the inframammary fold is the same with the previous description. (chapter 14, page 119.) (Fig. 14-1)
    The manual fixation is shown in (Fig. 14-2, 3).

(2) Implant selection

Surgeons should consider the breast footprint for implant selection. Breast width should be determined first. Then, volume should be considered. An implant with lighter weight than the mastectomy specimen is usually appropriate. In the author's opinion, a slightly bigger implant is better for the prepectoral technique than subpectoral technique because the ADM, which establishes the superficial envelope of the implant, is thinner than the pectoralis muscle in the

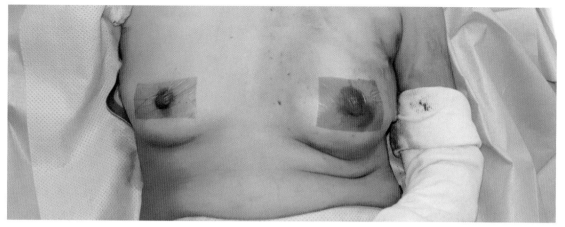

Fig. 14-1. Immediate postoperative image after breast implant sizer insertion. Inframammary fold (IMF) is descended to caudal direction. In this case, IMF correction is necessary

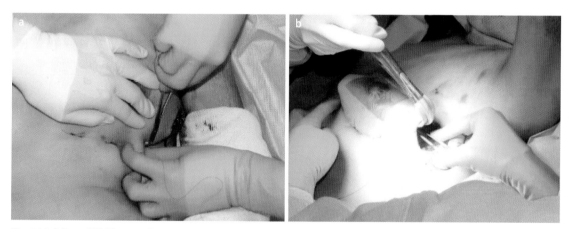

Fig. 14-2. Manual IMF correction

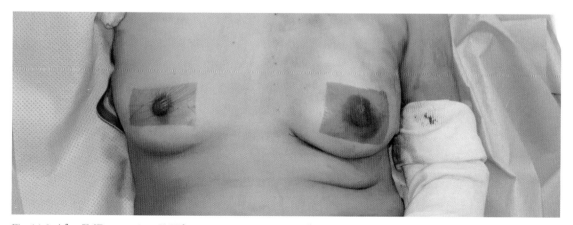

Fig. 14-3. After IMF correction. IMF becomes more symmetrical

subpectoral technique.

(3) Patient position

The position is the same as those in other breast prosthetic reconstructions. The arm at the operative side is fully abducted and fixed. The patient's body is tilted slightly to the non-operative side.

(4) Wrapping permanent implant

ADM with sufficient surface area should be used for wrapping the implant. Rupturing sutures around the ADM should be minimized in this step. However, ADM is not sufficient for full coverage of the permanent implant in some cases. The author (SYS) has developed a method of ADM coverage when ADM is not sufficient for wrapping. If ADM is not sufficient for full coverage, the whole anterior surface of the implant and posterior surface of the ptotic area of the breast should be covered. The Figure shows our method (Fig. 14-4).

(5) Pocket preparation

To minimize infection, the author (SYS) irrigates the pocket with triple antibiotics (for gram positive, gram negative, and anaerobes) (Fig. 14-5). Bleeding control is performed after the irrigation.

(6) Placement of drains

The author (SYS) prefers one drain at the inframammary fold and the other for the axilla and cephalic margin of the wrapped implant.

(7) Introduction of permanent implant

The wrapped implant is introduced into the pocket using a hyaluronic acid-coated funnel to protect the stitches of the ADM around the implant (Fig. 14-6).

(8) Closure of skin

A. Closure of the skin is described in chapter 13, page 113-114.

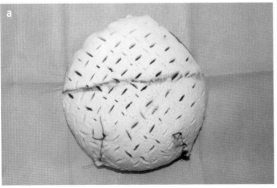
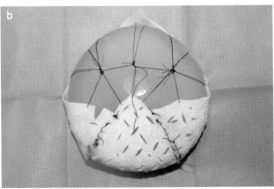

Fig. 14-4. A wrapping method for insufficient ADM.
a. The anterior side of the implant.
b. The posterior side of the implant

(9) Postoperative care

Postoperative care with elastic bandage and NO ointments is described in the chapter 14, page. 118.

Drain tubes are removed when the amount of drainage per day is consistently less than 30 cc.

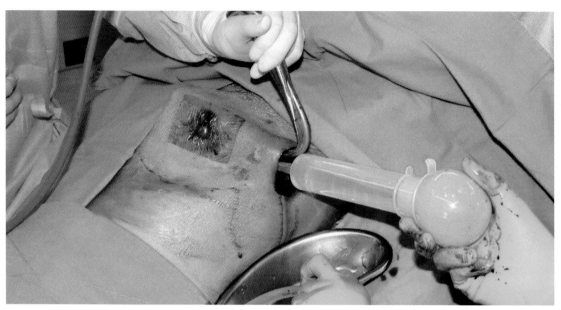

Fig. 14-5. Irrigation of the pocket with antibiotic solutions

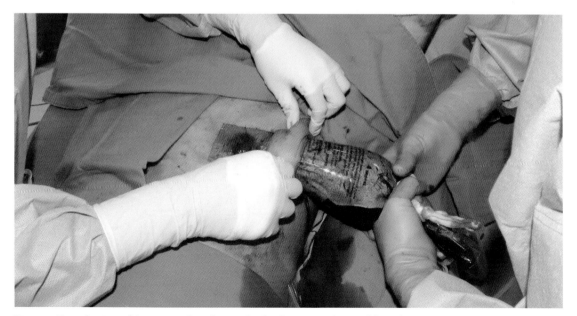

Fig. 14-6. Introduction of the wrapped implant with a hyaluronic acid-coated funnel

REFERENCES

1. Salzberg CA. Direct-to-implant breast reconstruction. Clinics in plastic surgery. 2012;39(2):119-26.

2. Colwell AS. Direct-to-implant breast reconstruction. Gland surgery. 2012;1(3):139-41.

3. Gruber RP, Kahn RA, Lash H, Maser MR, Apfelberg DB, Laub DR. Breast reconstruction following mastectomy: a comparison of submuscular and subcutaneous techniques. Plastic & Reconstructive Surgery. 1981;67(3):312-7.

4. Breuing KH, Warren SM. Immediate bilateral breast reconstruction with implants and inferolateral AlloDerm slings. Annals of plastic surgery. 2005;55(3):232-9.

5. Woo A, Harless C, Jacobson SR. Revisiting an Old Place: Single-Surgeon Experience on Post-Mastectomy Subcutaneous Implant-Based Breast Reconstruction. The Breast Journal. 2017;23(5):545-53.

6. Sigalove S, Maxwell GP, Sigalove NM, Storm Dickerson TL, Pope N, Rice J, et al. Prepectoral Implant-Based Breast Reconstruction: Rationale, Indications, and Preliminary Results. Plastic & Reconstructive Surgery. 2017;139(2):287-94.

15. Postoperative Results of Immediate Prosthetic Reconsturction after RNSM

Seung Yong Song

Case 1: Subpectoral two-stage prosthetic breast reconstruction

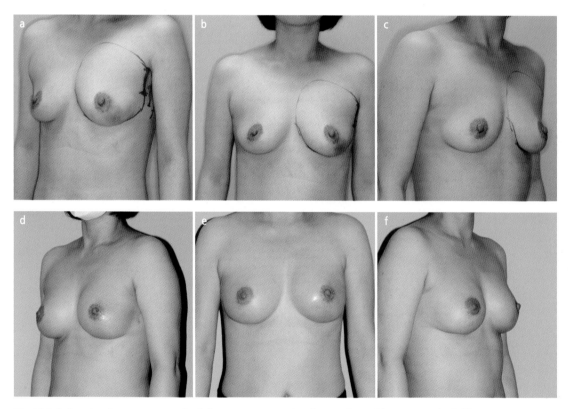

Fig. 15-1. Subpectoral two-stage prosthetic breast reconstruction for a patient with cancer in the left breast
a-c. Preoperative photographs
d-f. Postoperative 1 year, contralateral augmentation mammoplasty via axillary approach was performed

Case 2: Prepectoral two-stage prosthetic breast reconstruction

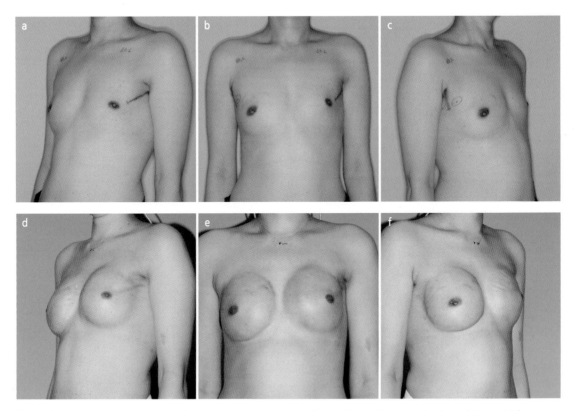

Fig. 15-2. Prepectoral two-stage prosthetic breast reconstruction for a patient with cancer in the right breast. The left breast was also reconstructed by the two-stage prepectoral method after prior conventional Nipple-Sparing mastectomy
a-c. Preoperative photographs
d-f. Postoperative 22 months

Case 3: Subpectoral DTI reconstruction

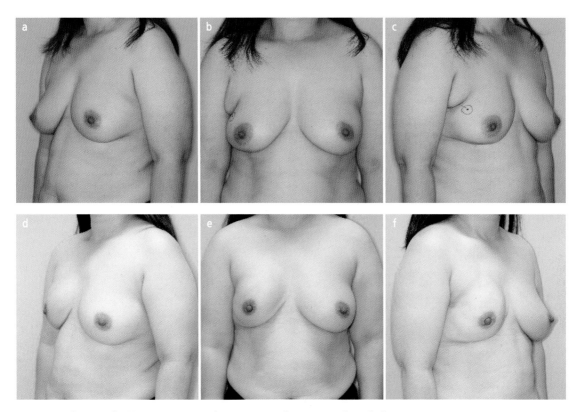

Fig. 15-3. Subpectoral DTI reconstruction for a patient with cancer in the right breast
a-c. Preoperative photographs
d-f. Postoperative 7 months

Case 4: Subpectoral DTI reconstruction

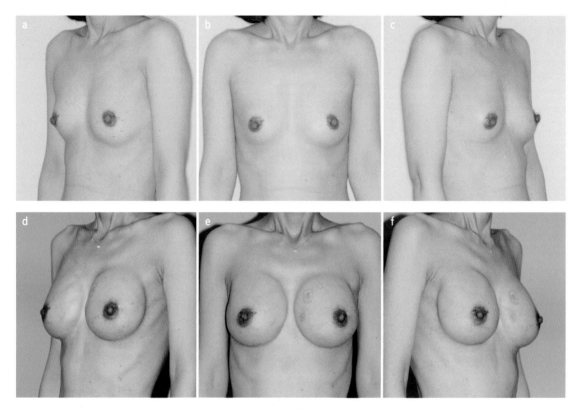

Fig. 15-4. Subpectoral DTI reconstruction for a patient with bilateral breast cancer
a-c. Preoperative photographs
d-f. Postoperative 1 year 6 months

Case 5: Prepectoral DTI reconstruction

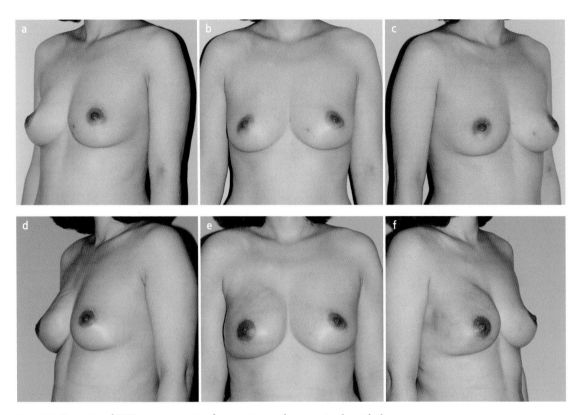

Fig. 15-5. Prepectoral DTI reconstruction for a patient with cancer in the right breast
a-c. Preoperative photographs
d-f. Postoperative 7 months

Case 6: Prepectoral DTI reconstruction

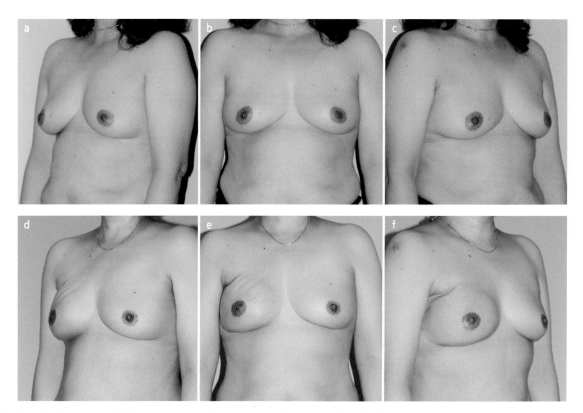

Fig. 15-6. Prepectoral DTI reconstruction for a patient with cancer in the right breast
a-c. Preoperative photographs
d-f. Postoperative 5 months

16. Postoperative Managements of Immediate Prosthetic Reconsturction after RNSM

Seung Yong Song

Secondary procedure

The cephalic area of the implant, the axilla, and the lateral chest wall are often depressed after implant insertion. If the patient complains of discomfort due to the depression in this area, a series of fat grafts can be helpful to alleviate these problems.

Complications

Hyperthermal injury

Intraoperative hyperthermal injury, including skin burn or blistering by an electrocautery, can occur. In prosthetic breast reconstruction, this can cause postoperative infection and delayed wound healing because of bacterial infection through the injury site. Active and appropriate treatments including early surgical repair should be considered in this condition.

Infection

Foreign bodies like the implant and large ADM are inserted during the prosthetic breast reconstruction. Therefore, infection of the implant site is one of the most serious complications after RNSM with reconstruction, which can even cause a failure of reconstruction.

In case of infection, patients complain of a heating sensation, erythema, and swelling of the wound with generalized fever and chills. If surgical site infection is suspected, early administration of empirical antibiotics is advocated. Appropriate bacterial culture of suspicious sites or serum should be taken. Immediate insertion of drains for seroma accumulation is recommended if indicated. Erythrocyte sedimentation rate (ESR) and C-reactive protein (CRP) can be checked to assess the degree of infection.

Although surgical site infection is difficult to manage in prosthetic breast reconstruction, proper treatments can salvage the implant and ADM.

Asymmetry

Asymmetry of the breasts is one of the major factors of patient dissatisfaction, especially in cases with DTI. Reconstructive surgeons should give special attention to the IMF position, pocket control, and proper selection of implants.

Skin depressions on axilla and upper chest wall

These phenomena are the results of discrepancy between the mastectomy area and the breast implant shape. This can be alleviated by multiple fat grafting procedures.

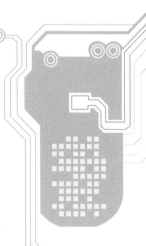

SECTION **05**

Robotic Immediate Breast Reconstruction Using Autologous Tissue

17. Introduction of Robotic Immediate Breast Reconstruction Using Autologous Tissue

Dong Won Lee and Hyung Seok Park

Reconstructive surgeons are relatively late adopters of minimally invasive surgery using endoscopy compared to surgeons in other fields, with the exception of some cosmetic procedures because of the importance of minimizing surgical scars. The reason is that reconstructive surgery generally does not use the natural body cavity like the abdominal or pelvic cavities, and most of them are targeted at the subcutaneous soft tissue. Specialized surgical techniques were necessary to maintain a satisfactory subcutaneous optical cavity.[1] This is similar to the case of robotic reconstructive surgery.

Breast reconstruction is one of the important processes for treatments for breast cancer. As all surgical techniques have improved, the purpose of breast reconstruction shifted from simply covering large volume defect after mastectomy to making breasts natural and aesthetically pleasing as well as reducing patient morbidity. Such a paradigm shift led to increased interest in minimally invasive surgery. Autologous tissues to supply added volume after mastectomy are commonly taken from the latissimus dorsi (LD) flap or the abdominal flap. The laparoscopic method for harvesting LD and rectus was first reported in the 1990s.[2,3] Recently, robotic harvest of LD flap and abdominal flap has also been developed by several plastic surgeons.[4-8] When the LD muscle is taken by robot, a reduced hospital stay as well as a smaller surgical scar are likely to follow. Also, robotic harvest of abdominal flap is thought to provide the reduction of donor site morbidity, minimizing the violation of donor site tissues. However, although these robotic techniques are showing feasibility, robotic surgery in breast reconstruction is not yet popular with plastic surgeons. In order to adopt the robotic technique in breast reconstruction, it is essential that a standard robotic procedure that is easily reproducible and provides advantages over the conventional method should be established.[9] To date, robotic surgery has already been applied to various surgical fields, and major advancements came with it. In this chapter, we describe the detailed techniques of robotic reconstructive breast surgery using autologous tissue.

REFERENCES

1. Hallock GG. A brief history of minimally invasive plastic surgery. Seminars in plastic surgery. 2008;22(1):5-7.

2. Fine NA, Orgill DP, Pribaz JJ. Early clinical experience in endoscopic-assisted muscle flap harvest. Annals of plastic surgery. 1994;33(5):465-9; discussion 9-72.

3. Bass LS, Karp NS, Benacquista T, Kasabian AK. Endoscopic harvest of the rectus abdominis free flap: balloon dissection in the fascial plane. Annals of plastic surgery. 1995;34(3):274-9; discussion 9-80.

4. Selber JC, Baumann DP, Holsinger FC. Robotic latissimus dorsi muscle harvest: a case series. Plastic and reconstructive surgery. 2012;129(6):1305-12.

5. Clemens MW, Kronowitz S, Selber JC. Robotic-assisted latissimus dorsi harvest in delayed-immediate breast reconstruction. Seminars in plastic surgery. 2014;28(1):20-5.

6. Chung JH, You HJ, Kim HS, Lee BI, Park SH, Yoon ES. A novel technique for robot assisted latissimus dorsi flap harvest. Journal of plastic, reconstructive & aesthetic surgery : JPRAS. 2015;68(7):966-72.

7. Gundlapalli VS, Ogunleye AA, Scott K, Wenzinger E, Ulm JP, Tavana L, et al. Robotic-assisted deep inferior epigastric artery perforator flap abdominal harvest for breast reconstruction: A case report. Microsurgery. 2018;38(6):702-5.

8. Selber JC. The Robotic DIEP Flap. Plastic and reconstructive surgery. 2020;145(2):340-3.

9. Donnely E, Griffin MF, Butler PE. Robotic Surgery: A Novel Approach for Breast Surgery and Reconstruction. Plastic and reconstructive surgery Global open. 2020;8(1):e2578.

18. Robotic Harvest of Latissimus Dorsi Flap

Dong Won Lee

Traditionally, harvesting of the LD flap needs a long incision, which leaves a long donor scar and may be an unpleasant burden to patients. Thus, there have been many attempts to lessen the scar using a minimally invasive approach. Robotic harvesting of the LD muscle was first performed by Selber.[1] He tested the feasibility in a cadaveric model and demonstrated the clinical application. Chung et al.[2] reported a different technique with gasless robotic harvest.

For harvesting LD muscle distributed in the large area of the back using laparoscopic approach, there is a major concern about reaching the medial border with a camera scope and dissectors. Since the muscle curves posteromedially to follow the curvature of the back, the rigid chest wall can restrict the manipulation of rigid laparoscopic instruments. The way to overcome this limitation can be found in flexible robotic arms. Furthermore, a recently introduced single-port robotic surgical system, da Vinci SP, provides flexible motion of the camera, which enables coverage of the whole surgical field of the LD flap.

Patient selection

LD flap harvested by robot has limited indications, given that skin flap is not included in the LD flap.[3] The robotic harvest of LD muscle should be considered in situations where only muscle, and not the skin flap island is needed. These are the indications for robotic breast reconstruction using the LD flap: (1) breast reconstruction with LD muscle plus fat graft in very small breasts, (2) oncoplastic surgery with LD muscle flap after breast conserving surgery, (3) implant-based, delayed-immediate reconstruction of the radiated breast,[4] (4) lower pole coverage instead of acellular dermal matrix in prosthetic reconstruction, and (5) Poland syndrome in a male breast.

Among those indications, the techniques for breast reconstruction with LD muscle plus fat graft using a single port robotic surgical system in very small breasts after robot-assisted Nipple-Sparing mastectomy is shown below.

REFERENCES

1. Selber JC, Baumann DP, Holsinger FC. Robotic latissimus dorsi muscle harvest: a case series. Plastic and reconstructive surgery. 2012;129(6):1305-12.

2. Chung JH, You HJ, Kim HS, Lee BI, Park SH, Yoon ES. A novel technique for robot assisted latissimus dorsi flap harvest. Journal of plastic, reconstructive & aesthetic surgery : JPRAS. 2015;68(7):966-72.

3. Chang HP, Fan KL, Song SY, Lee DW. The traditional versus endoscopic-assisted latissimus dorsi harvest in oncoplastic surgery: A long term comparison of breast volume, aesthetics, and donor site outcomes. Asian journal of surgery. 2020;43(12):1165-71.

4. Clemens MW, Kronowitz S, Selber JC. Robotic-assisted latissimus dorsi harvest in delayed-immediate breast reconstruction. Seminars in plastic surgery. 2014;28(1): 20-5.

19. Step-by-Step Procedures for Latissimus Dorsi Flap

Dong Won Lee

Pedicle dissection

First, after mastectomy, the anterior border of the LD muscle is identified via the axillary incision made by a breast surgeon. The thoracodorsal branch, which originates from the subscapular vessel, runs from the axilla along the anterior border of the latissimus dorsi muscle and enters into the deep surface of the LD muscle. The thoracodorsal nerve, which courses with thoracodorsal vessel, is ligated to prevent unwanted movement of a reconstructed breast. However, some surgeons prefer to leave the nerve uncut in order to maintain muscle volume with the expectation that transferred LD muscle will not atrophy.

Patient position

The patient is placed in the lateral decubitus position. The patient's ipsilateral arm is positioned below her shoulder to prevent collision with the robotic arms. The operative field is prepared to open the affected breast and back between the scapula and iliac crest.

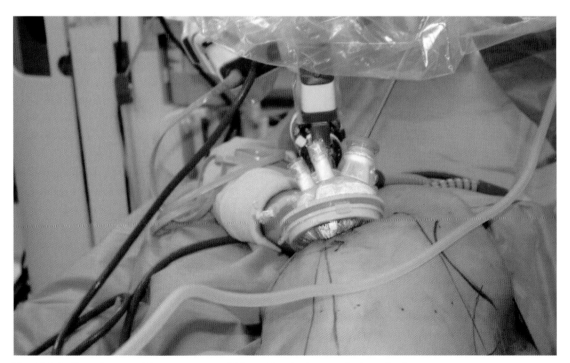

Fig. 19-1. Ipsilateral arm position to prevent collision with robotic arms during robotic surgery

Design

The patient is prepared and draped in the standard fashion. The significant anatomical landmarks are marked: the posterior axillary line, the posterior midline, and the inferior tip of the scapula. The LD muscle to be harvested is outlined. It is recommended that the lateral margin of the LD muscle to be harvested is slightly medial to the posterior axillary line to allow unrestricted and comfortable motion of the robotic arms. Since the robotic arms of the single-port robotic surgical system have a reach of 24 cm from the port, the inferior and medial margin of the LD muscle to be harvested should be within this range. Although there is a limitation of reach distance of the robotic arms, most of the LD muscle can be obtained.

Creation of working space

A subcutaneous space anterior and posterior to the anterior border of the muscle is dissected using a long-tip electrocautery and a lighted retractor in order to create working space for placement of a single port device and initiation of robotic surgery. Manual dissection to create the half-circle working space with a radius of 10-15 cm from the incision is sufficient.

Attachment of a single port device and port placement

When using a single port robotic surgical system, the axillary incision made by the breast surgeon is used for robotic dissection of LD muscle, and no additional incision is required. Prior to port placement, a single port device is attached to the axillary incision. There are currently several commercial devices (refer to Table 8-2). A single port device can be chosen according to the surgeon's preference.

After the application of a wound protector, a port is attached. For the harvest of LD muscle, two steps are needed: the first is

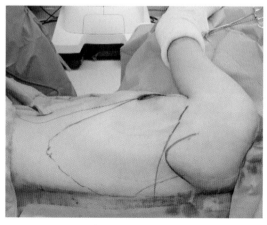

Fig. 19-2. Design of important anatomical landmarks and latissimus dorsi muscle to be harvested

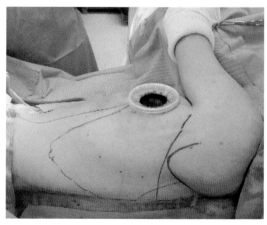

Fig. 19-3. Attachment of a single port device (UNI-PORT)

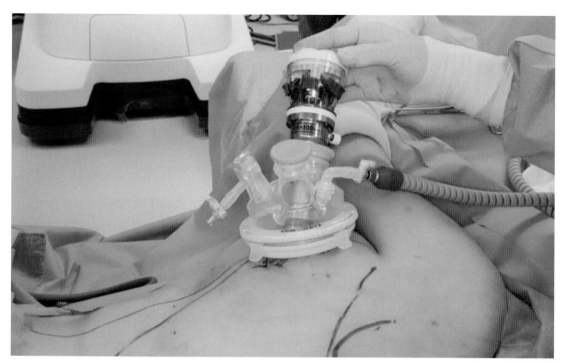

Fig. 19-4. Port placement into undersurface of latissimus dorsi muscle

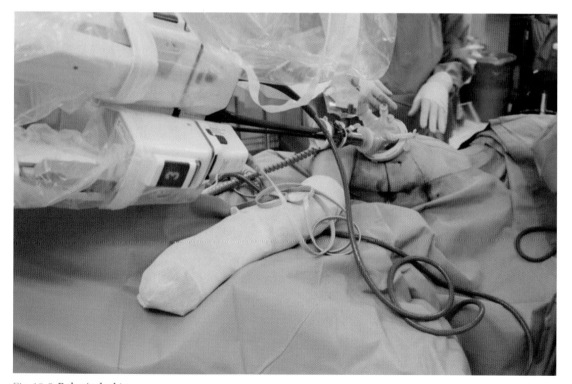

Fig. 19-5. Robotic docking

dissection of the LD undersurface, and the second is dissection of the superficial surface of the LD muscle. If done in reverse, it would be hard to maintain actual working space with gas insufflation when dissecting the undersurface of the LD muscle in the second step. This is because the gas tends to flow into the superficial space of LD muscle, which would be made in the first step. Accordingly, the author recommends dissection of the LD undersurface first. The tip of the cannula is placed under the LD muscle at the first step. CO_2 insufflation is maintained at 8 mmHg.

Robotic docking

The ports are docked to the robotic arms. The axis of the instrument arms is directed toward the T12 vertebra from the axillary incision. Robotic instruments include the da Vinci SP® Cadiere grasping forceps (Intuitive Surgical Inc., Sunnyvale, CA) for the first instrument drive and the da Vinci SP® monopolar curved scissors (Intuitive Surgical Inc., Sunnyvale, CA) for the third instrument drive. The camera is docked on the upper side of the instrument drive, thus facilitating the vision of the camera even in the medial part of the breast where the rigid curved chest wall can restrict the visual field.

Robotic dissection

Submuscular dissection is performed. Perforating vessels within the submuscular plane are carefully coagulated with monopolar

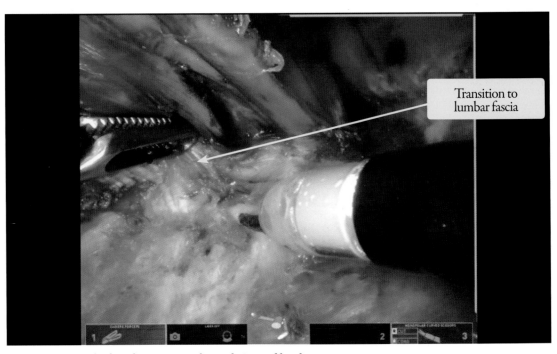

Fig. 19-6. Cutting the fascial transition at the predesignated borders

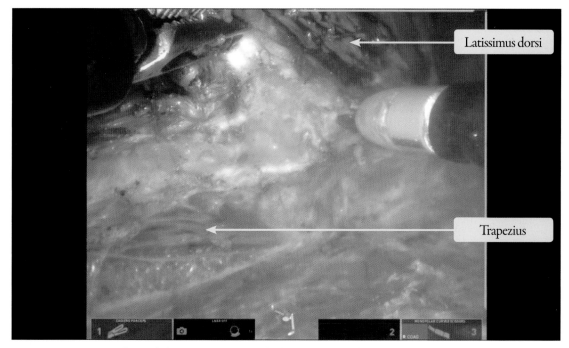

Fig. 19-7. Dissection at the medial extreme separating the latissimus dorsi from the trapezius

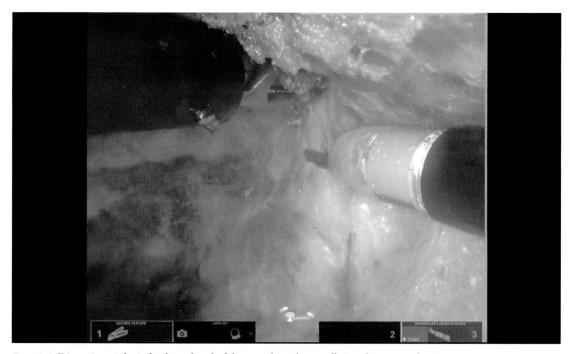

Fig. 19-8. Dissection at the inferolateral end of the muscle without collisions between robotic arms

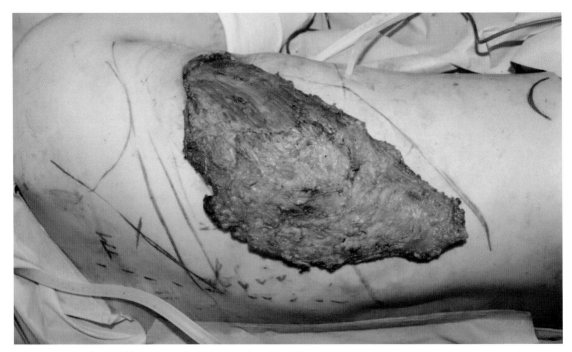

Fig. 19-9. Completion of harvesting the latissimus dorsi muscle

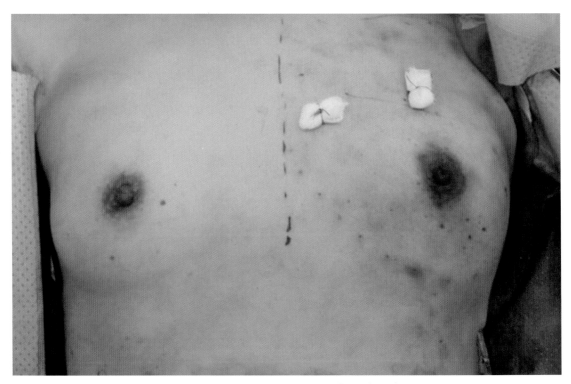

Fig. 19-10. Breast reconstruction with the latissimus dorsi muscle plus fat grafting

predesigned borders is cut, and dissection is continued until the fat layer is exposed. Once submuscular dissection is complete, the port's position is moved to the subcutaneous plane. Undocking is not necessary but may facilitate changing port placement. Dissection of the superficial surface of the muscle is performed. When subcutaneous dissection reaches the predesignated borders, subcutaneous space is connected together with submuscular space and the muscle is disinserted.

When using multiport robot systems, the robotic arms and camera become parallel and conflict with one another at the medial and lateral extremes of the dissection.[1] But a single port robot system can overcome this limitation by minimizing collisions between the robotic arms. Moreover, it is helpful to use the cobra position of the camera because all structures can be seen without blind spots, especially in the medial part where the curvature of the back can restrict the visual field.

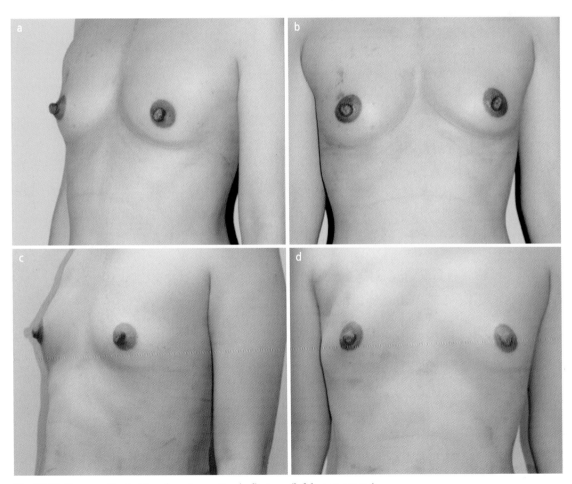

Fig. 19-11. Preoperative (a,b) and postoperative (c,d) views (left breast cancer)

Undocking and completion of muscle harvest

The robot is undocked, and the single port device is also detached. If there is any remaining attachment when extracting the LD muscle, it usually exists around the teres major muscle and the inferior tip of the scapula. The attachment can be easily divided using a long-tip electrocautery and a lighted retractor. The totally separated LD muscle is transferred into the mastectomy pocket.

Breast reconstruction with the latissimus dorsi muscle and fat grafting

The patient's position is changed to supine with the arm abducted. The volume of muscles only is not sufficient for breast reconstruction, even in small breasts. Fat grafting or implant insertion is required for accomplishing a balanced breast. In the case of fat grafting, fat is harvested from the patient's abdomen or thigh. Autologous fat is grafted into the LD muscle and pectoralis major muscle. The upper pole of the breast is augmented with fat in pectoralis major, and the lower pole is formed mainly by LD muscle plus grafted fat. The LD flap is fixed using pull-out sutures. This method can restore the breast volume up to 150–200 ml.

REFERENCES

1. Selber JC, Baumann DP, Holsinger FC. Robotic latissimus dorsi muscle harvest: a case series. Plastic and reconstructive surgery. 2012;129(6):1305-12.

20. Robotic Harvest of Deep Inferior Epigastric Perforator Flap

Dong Won Lee

Autologous breast reconstruction using abdominal tissue has been developed in the direction of decreasing the donor site morbidity. First, the pedicled transverse rectus abdominis musculocutaneous (TRAM) flap was introduced in 1982,[1] soon followed by the free TRAM flap. As a next step, muscle-sparing free TRAM flap was presented with reduced donor site morbidity by minimizing the harvest of the anterior rectus fascia. Since the deep inferior epigastric perforator (DIEP) flap was introduced early in the 1990s,[2, 3] it increasingly gained popularity, and currently is the most common perforator flap for microsurgical breast reconstruction. Rectus abdominis muscle and anterior rectus fascia are not included in the DIEP flap, and can be preserved at the donor site. With the advent of surgical techniques, damage of donor site has been minimized, and thus the donor site morbidity is expected to be reduced. However, even during the DIEP flap elevation, violation to the anterior rectus sheath, rectus muscle and motor nerves is inevitable. In order to expose the deep inferior epigastric artery, dissection, splitting, and traction of the upper structures above the pedicle are required. All of these procedures may cause donor site morbidity. The way to overcome these limitations can be found in minimally invasive surgeries such as the robotic approach.

Robotic harvest of rectus[4] muscle was first introduced by Patel et al.[4] who used a da Vinci surgical robot system with transabdominal preperitoneal (TAPP) approach. Afterward, Gundlapalli and his colleague[5] reported one case of robotic DIEP flap harvest for breast reconstruction with the TAPP approach. Hivelin et al.[4] published a report about minimally invasive dissected DIEP flap using the totally extraperitoneal (TEP) approach with laparoscopic devices, not robotic. While the TAPP approach is carried out using the peritoneal cavity, the TEP approach uses the preperitoneal space, which is not only narrow but also difficult to convert to an actual space from a potential space. Thus, the TEP approach has a long and steep learning curve. The single-port surgical robot system is recently updated and optimized to narrow surgical spaces. Procedures using this system can be a feasible option to harvest the DIEP flap using the TEP approach with a shorter learning curve. Among various techniques, robotic harvest of the DIEP flap with the TEP approach using the single port robot system for breast reconstruction is shown below.

Patient selection

During harvesting of the DIEP flap, the robotic surgical system is applied in the dissection of the pedicle coursing under the rectus muscle. The longer the length of the pedicle underneath the rectus muscle is, the more suitable the patient is. On the other hand, the advantage is reduced when the intramuscular course is long or when more than one perforator is needed. The ideal indication is a patient who has a pedicle with one large perforator and a short intramuscular course.

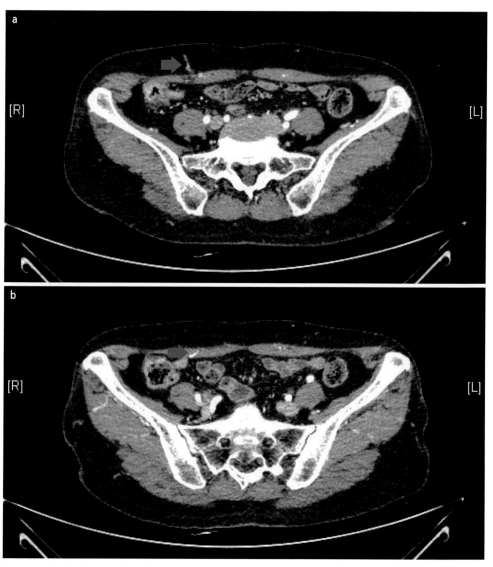

Fig. 20-1. Ideal indication for robotic DIEP harvest: one large perforator and a short intramuscular course

REFERENCES

1. Hartrampf CR, Scheflan M, Black PW. Breast reconstruction with a transverse abdominal island flap. Plastic and reconstructive surgery. 1982;69(2):216-25.

2. Koshima I, Soeda S. Inferior epigastric artery skin flaps without rectus abdominis muscle. British journal of plastic surgery. 1989;42(6):645-8.

3. Allen RJ, Treece P. Deep inferior epigastric perforator flap for breast reconstruction. Annals of plastic surgery. 1994;32(1):32-8.

4. Patel NV, Pedersen JC. Robotic harvest of the rectus abdominis muscle: a preclinical investigation and case report. Journal of reconstructive microsurgery. 2012;28(7):477-80.

5. Gundlapalli VS, Ogunleye AA, Scott K, Wenzinger E, Ulm JP, Tavana L, et al. Robotic-assisted deep inferior epigastric artery perforator flap abdominal harvest for breast reconstruction: A case report. Microsurgery. 2018;38(6):702-5.

21. Step-by-Step Procedures for Deep Inferior Epigastric Perforator Flap

Dong Won Lee

Pedicle selection

The course of the deep inferior epigastric vessels needs to be reviewed with computed tomographic angiography (CTA) prior to surgery. If the patient is proven to have a longer intramuscular course than submuscular course in CTA, robotic harvest would not be recommended. In preoperative CTA, appropriate perforators are selected, and intramuscular and submuscular course are confirmed.

Pedicle dissection from the preselected perforator before the intramuscular course ends

The abdominal flap is elevated with the conventional method. Dissection of the preselected perforators is performed with small fascial incision until just before the intramuscular course ends. The reason not to penetrate the rectus muscle is to prevent the leakage of carbon dioxide when insufflating CO_2 into the working space.

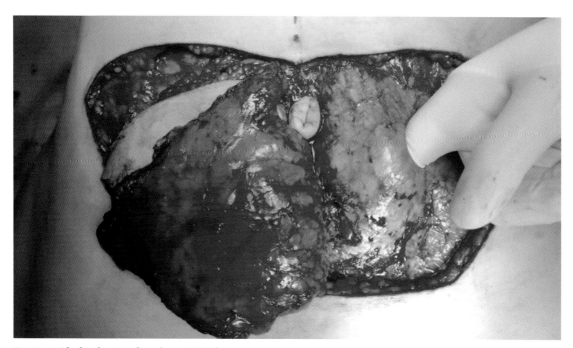

Fig. 21-1. Ideal indication for robotic DIEP harvest

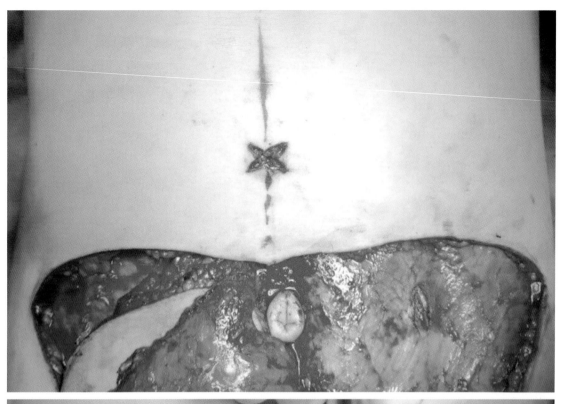

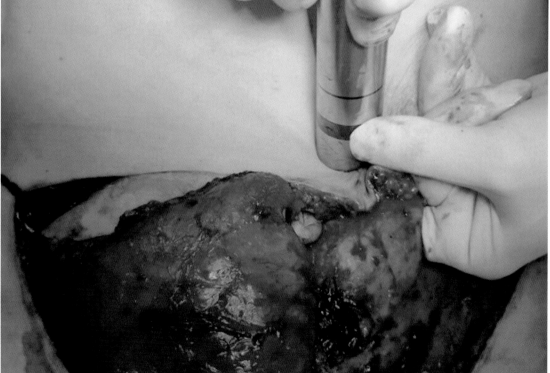

Fig. 21-2. Port incision and insertion into the preperitoneal space

Creation of preperitoneal space

Before docking the robot, a potential preperitoneal space is converted to an actual space to facilitate robotic dissection. A small vertical incision is made on the linea semilunaris. Through this incision, preperitoneal blunt dissection is performed with the surgeon's finger or a balloon device (OMS-PDB1000, Covidien, Dublin, Ireland) to create the actual working space without any injury in the muscle or nerve.

Port placement

Two 2 cm-skin incisions are made in a cross shape at the site of the new umbilicus for the insertion of a 2.5 cm-diameter single port. The port is placed directly through the fascia into the preperitoneal space with the assistance of the index finger to avoid damage to the peritoneum by the port. The fascial incision at linea semilunaris is repaired to prevent gas leakage, and carbon dioxide is insufflated at 8 mmHg.

Robotic docking and patient position

When docking the robot, the operation table is put in a Trendelenburg position to prevent the robotic arms from colliding with the patient's head or chest. The axis

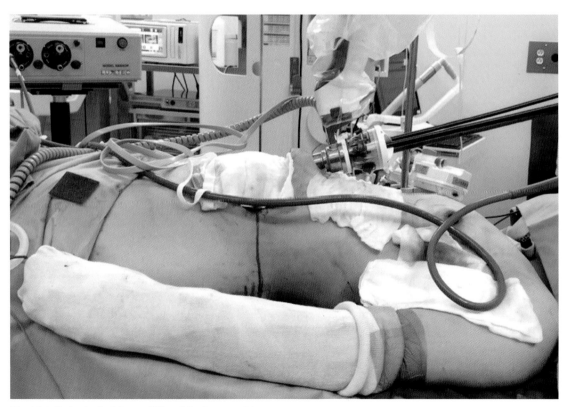

Fig. 21-3. Robotic docking and Trendelenburg position

of the instrument arms is aligned towards the external iliac artery in the inguinal area. The da Vinci SP® Maryland bipolar forceps (Intuitive Surgical Inc., Sunnyvale, CA) are mounted in the first and second instrument drives on both sides, and the da Vinci SP® monopolar curved scissors (Intuitive Surgical Inc., Sunnyvale, CA) are mounted in the third drive on the right side. The camera is docked on the lowest part of the port, and the other arms are docked on the upper sides, thus preventing the robotic arms from getting caught by the arcuate line.

Robotic harvest

After docking the robot arms, pedicle dissection under the rectus muscle is performed. Since there is no posterior rectus sheath below the arcuate line, that area is more expandable, and a wider view of the preperitoneal cavity facilitates robotic surgery. The camera, set in a cobra position, allows all structures around the pedicle to be clearly visible. All collateral vascular branches are ligated to free the pedicle. The pedicle is clipped near the origin and divided.

Undocking and completion of flap elevation

The robot is undocked, and remaining attachments from the intramuscular part are divided under direct vision. Finally, the pedicle is pulled out through the fascial incision. After robotic procedures, the surgery proceeds in the standard fashion.

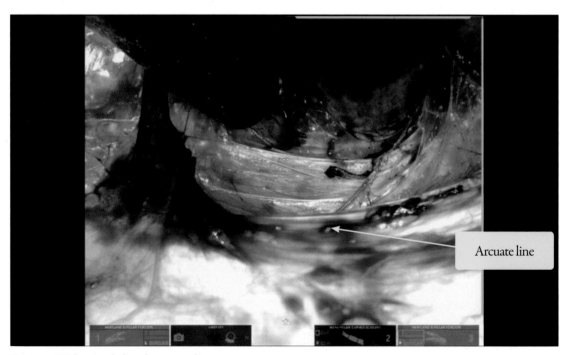

Fig. 21-4. Wider view below the arcuate line

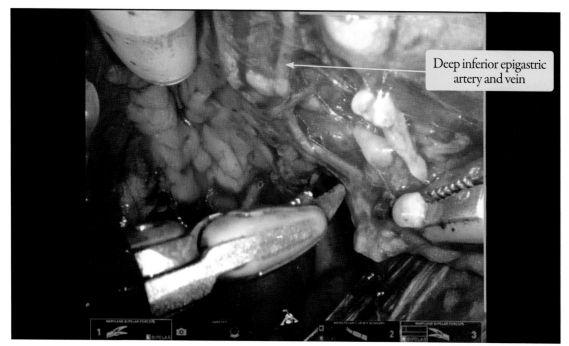

Fig. 21-5. Ligation of collateral branch

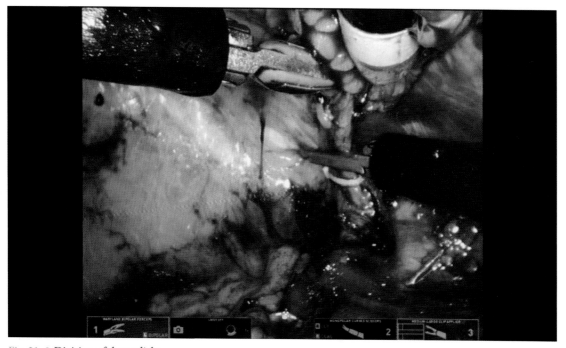

Fig. 21-6. Division of the pedicle

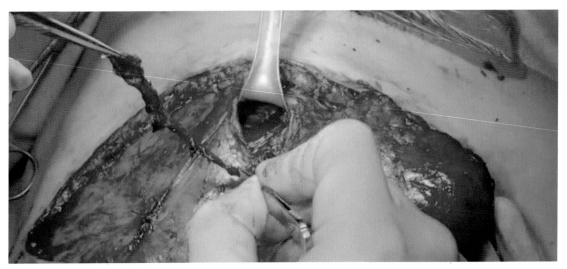

Fig. 21-7. The pedicle pulled out through the small fascial incision

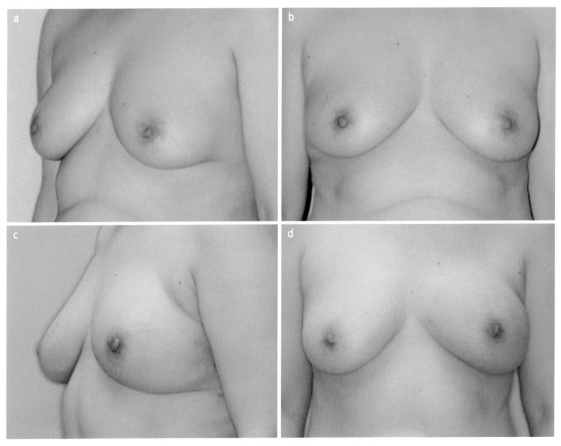

Fig. 21-8. a, b. Preoperative views (breast cancer in the left), c, d. Postoperative views,
Figure C shows the incision after RNSM and Figure D shows good cosmetic result after RNSM.

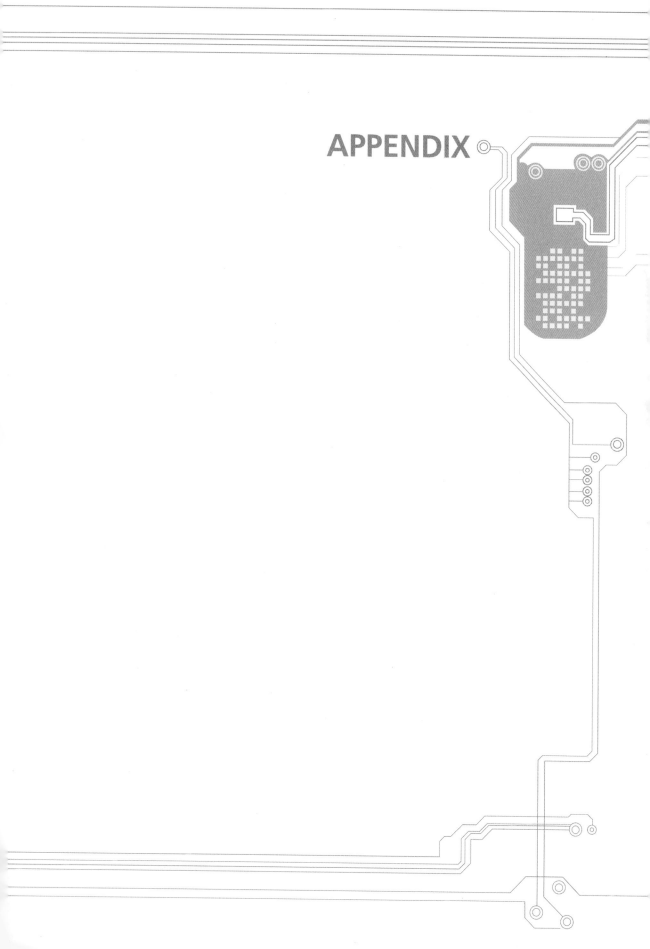

APPENDIX

Standard Operating Procedure Ver. 1.0 for the Gas-Inflated Robotic Nipple-Sparing Mastectomy Using a Multiport Robotic Surgical System (da Vinci Xi)

Haemin Lee, Jeea Lee, and Hyung Seok Park

Procedure	Details
1. Position 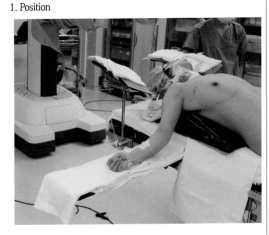	Move the patient to the edge of the table of the surgery, and keep the torso lifted with a sponge backrest shoulder pad. 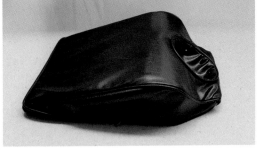 Spread the arms and hang the armrest on the side so that it can be lifted above the head later (Support the gel–pad properly to prevent the occurrence of sores). Adjust the position of the armrest or apply a protective band to the patient's face to prevent the armrest from hitting the patient's face. 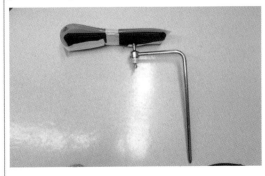

Precautions	Checklist
Place sufficient pads or sheets below the head to keep the cervical spine and airway at an adequate posture. (This is to prevent the robot arm from being caught by the armboard or the table. For the same reason, remove the pad from the arm board to let the arm drop at an angle where the elbow is slightly bent.) 	☐ Has the backrest shoulder pad been installed? ☐ Has the ipsilateral border of the patient's torso been placed at the edge of the table? ☐ Has the armboard been installed? ☐ Is the airway being maintained? ☐ Is the neck NOT over-extended?

Procedure	Details
2. Draping	Unfold the armboard at an angle of 90°, and cover with a legging drape. The rest of the procedure is similar with that of conventional mastectomy.

Precautions	Checklist
Cover the armboard and the legging drape to prevent from contamination.	☐ Has the draping been completed without contamination?

Procedure	Details
3. Border marking and dye injection 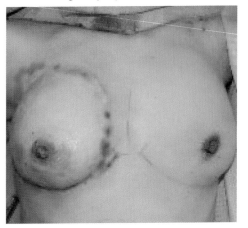	Using vital blue dye is helpful to perform sentinel lymph node biopsy (SLNB) and border marking. Carefully inject the blue dye (i.e. indigo carmine, isosulfan blue) around the nipple–areolar complex (NAC) and into the breast border at intervals of one o'clock on a 12 o'clock basis. 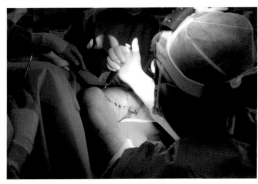
4. Incision 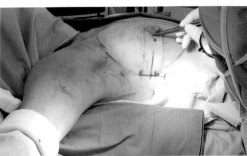 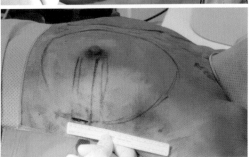 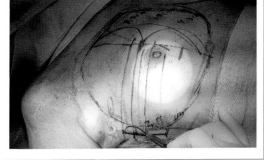	From the chair position, adjust the table to the level of the operator's eye level and tilt the surgical side up by the elevation (15~20 degrees) 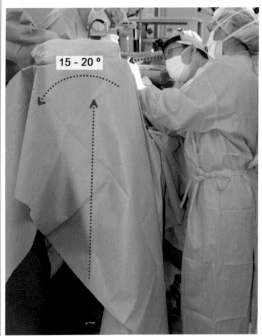 The incision size begins with a multiport of 4 cm (adjusted to the port size) and adjusts the size to 2.5–6 cm considering the breast size. Incision is made in the lateral side of NAC between mid and anterior axilla. It is also possible to put an incision on the lateral side adjusting the midpoint of vertical length in the breast (Red Arrow in the figure), not at NAC level.

Precautions	Checklist
Inserting a thick syringe has risks of developing pneumothorax. Therefore, it is NOT recommended. Thin and short 1cc syringe (26G) is recommended. SLNB can be performed by a radioisotope method. Please, be careful of a rare event of anaphylaxis to blue dye.	☐ Has the injection been done with a 26 gauge needle for sentinel and border marking? 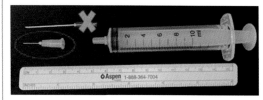

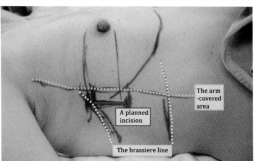

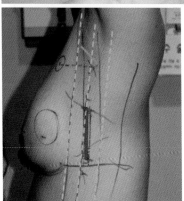

☐ Has the table been elevated and tilted?

☐ Has the hot−uptake area in the axilla been identified with a gamma probe before surgery?

☐ Have the location and size of the incision been estimated to perform sentinel node biopsy?

☐ Has the incision size been checked and documented with a ruler before incision?

Before the surgery, it is necessary to draw the incision line considering the brassiere line and the place where she naturally lowers her arms while the patient is wearing her bra. If possible, choose where the incision line is covered by the arms and the bra.

Incision is made using a gamma probe before surgery to find out where to implement the SLNB and to check the distance from the incision.

Procedure	Details
5. Sentinel lymph node biopsy	After Incision, perform SLNB first. 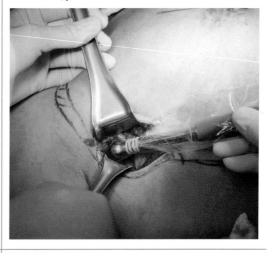
6. Making working space 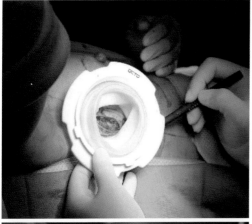 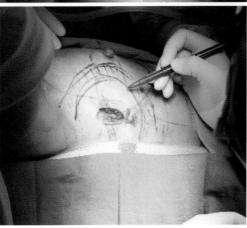	Draw an imaginary semicircular line of the working space that is 1.5–2 times as large as the wound protector's diameter first and then make the skin flap of the working space manually. 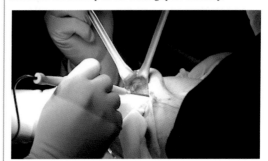

Precautions	Checklist
	☐ Has the SLNB been successful?
The lateral side of the working space is extended towards the superior and inferior pole direction	☐ Has the working space been made towards the nipple and the area under the imaginary semicircle? ☐ Has the working space been made towards the upper direction (to the 12−1 o'clock direction in the left breast) and has the lateral border of the pectoralis major muscle been identified? ☐ Has the working space been made towards the lower direction (to the 5 o'clock direction in the left breast), and has the lateral border of the pectoralis major muscle been identified?

Procedure	Details
7. Dissection of the retromammary space and checking the working space 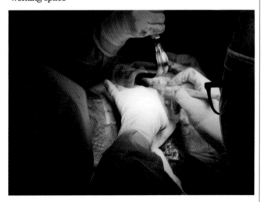	Find the retromammary space from the beginning of the breast lateral border. 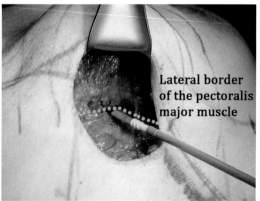 The retromammary space is almost dissected before docking. An assistant stands on the opposite side and lifts the breast with fiber−optic retractors. ▼ fiber−optic retractors 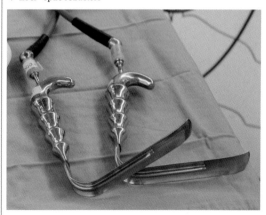 Proceed as much dissection as possible to the upper, inner, and lower borders. If possible, proceed to the point where the injected dye is visible. 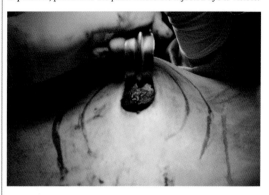

Precautions	Checklist
Please ensure that your dissection plane is the retromammary space, not the inter-pectoral space. Sometimes, beginners confuse this dissection plane. It is easier to dock after dissecting the border from the axillary tail to the inferior pole located at a 6 o'clock direction in the breast. This area may not be easy to access with a multiport robot system.	☐ Has the retromammary space just above the pectoralis muscle been identified? ☐ Has the retromammary space of the upper, inner, and lower borders been dissected as much as possible?

Procedure	Details
8. Tumescent injection	Inject 200–400 cc of the tumescent solution (Mix with 5% dextrose water or normal saline + epinephrine 1 ample + lidocaine 1 ample) evenly under the flap using the long needle or Veress needle ▼ long needle 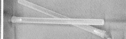 ▼ Veress needle 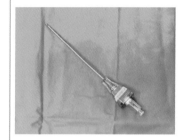
9. Tunneling or superficial layer dissection 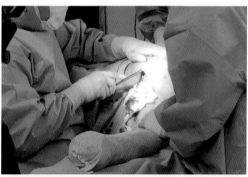 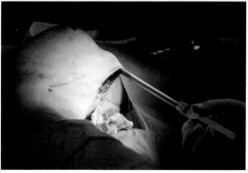	Proceed the tunneling or blunt dissection under the flap using Metzenbaum scissors or a vascular tunneler. 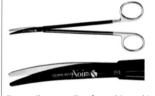 Proceeding tunneling from side to side of the NAC, not directly below NAC, can help to guide you to find the nipple after docking. After finishing tunneling, gently squeeze the solution out from the breast. 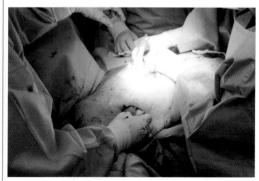

Precautions	Checklist
	☐ Has the tumescent solution mixing been done properly? ☐ Was the tumescent solution injected evenly?
Be careful not to cut the flap too thin. Be careful not to squeeze too much to prevent squeezing tumor.	☐ Have you approached to the end of the breast border using the tunneling technique by the scissors or a vascular tunneler? ☐ Has it been tunneled on both sides of the nipple-areolar complex? ☐ Is the thickness of the flap of the tunneling appropriate?

Procedure	Details
10. Single port device insertion and cannula placement 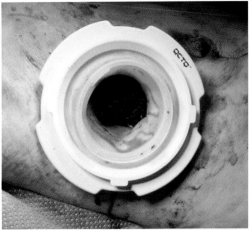 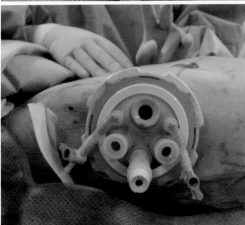 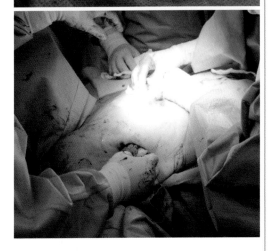	Attach a single port device (i.e. UNI-PORT) to the incision and insert cannulas into the port. The camera uses the largest connection part of the device, and the acting robotic arms are located on each side of the cannula of the camera. Connect a CO_2 gas valve and inject CO_2 with the pressure of 8 mmHg, flow 8–10 ml. 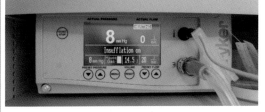 ▼ UNI-PORT 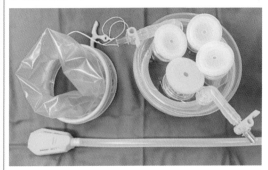

Precautions	Checklist
When using OCTO™ port, to adjust the cannula size, remove white plastic caps. 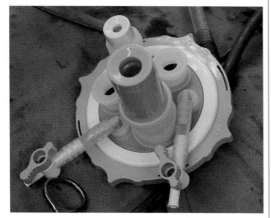	☐ When using OCTO™ port, are white plastic caps removed? ☐ Is the wound protector of the single port device properly inserted? ☐ Is there enough distance between the external ring of the wound protector and working space? (about 5–10 cm apart) ☐ Has the biggest camera port (i.e. the blue connection part of OCTO™ port, the green connection part of UNI−PORT) been located above and the three white ports below? ☐ Has each robot cannula been secured so that the inner thick line of the remote center is located within the connection part? ☐ Is the pressure and flow of the gas appropriate? (8 mmHg, 8–10 ml) ☐ Is the gas Inflation successful? Is the flap filled with gas to allow good distention?

Procedure	Details
11. Robot docking 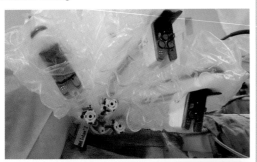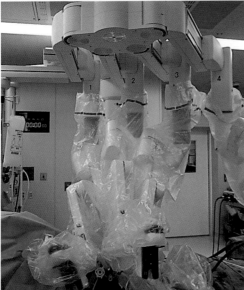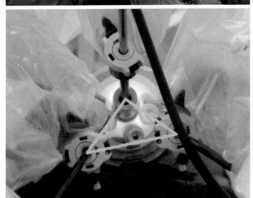	Fold and attach the armrest to the table or detach the armrest before docking. Fix the arm or put it on the armrest above the head. Dock with the robot. In the case of multiport systems, the author prefers that the green cross in the control center is adjusted from the camera port to the middle thickness line in the remote center of the trocar, without the targeting 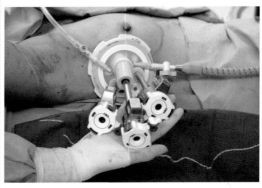 Place the green transverse line of the control center in a straight line at the nipple First, set up the camera in the camera connection part of the single port device. Place Prograsp forceps for the left hand and monoploar scissors for the right hand Check the instruments of both hands are properly inserted 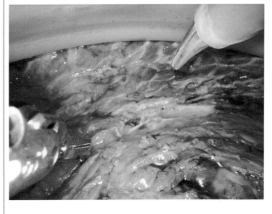

Precautions	Checklist
When the patient cart comes in, beware not to collide with the patient's head or body. When beginning, keep the camera up to 30˚. This will help with flap developing. 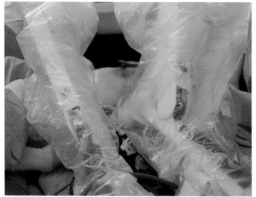 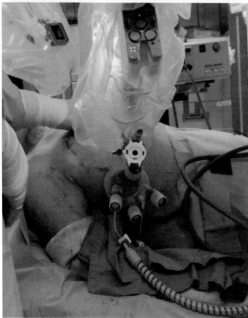	☐ Is the green cross of the control center set on the middle thick line of the cannula? ☐ Is the green transverse line of the control center placed straight to meet the center of the nipple? ☐ Are there no foreign bodies (such as tape, gauze etc.) inside the working space before docking? ☐ Is the camera installed in an angle of 30˚ upward? ☐ Have you checked on the monitor whether the equipment in both hands are properly installed?

Procedure	Details
12. Flap dissection toward the nipple	Move the camera and find the tunneling site of the subcutaneous flap. Carry out flap dissection toward the nipple. When doing so, an assistant on the field must carefully check to see no flap injuries are being made. 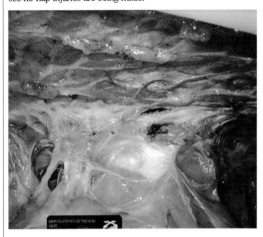 ▼ View of an assistant 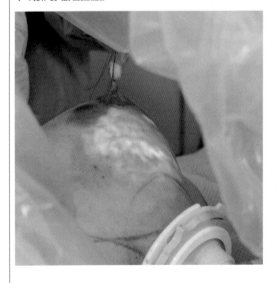

Precautions	Checklist
When moving the camera, pull the internal ring of the wound protector as upward as possible and insert the camera into the working space. When doing so, you are able to see the tunneling by scissors or a tunneler. Adjust and make the thickness of the flap using this thickness as reference.	☐ Has the subcutaneous flap been checked by moving the camera? ☐ Do you have a clear view of the tunneling site after insertion of the camera? The camera should show the tunneling of the subcutaneous flap, not the retromammary space.

Procedure	Details
13. Nipple–areolar complex margin biopsy	If the fibrotic white tissue of the NAC is visible, suture the outside of the nipple and pull it. Pull the nipple upwards while doing the dissection the both sides and the bottom tissue of the NAC

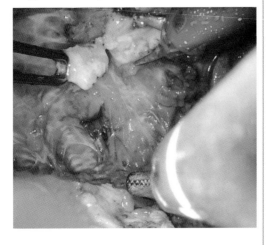

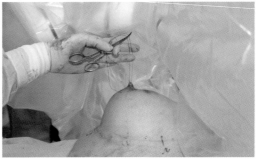

When the subareolar tissue is all exposed, verify the exact location of the nipple core while the assistant is pressing the nipple in the field.

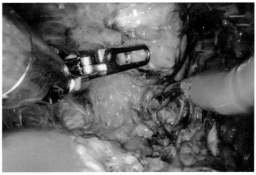

Check the position of the nipple core and hold it with grasper. After holding the nipple, the assistant can control pressing the nipple. While holding the core, use the right scissors for coring dissection in order to obtain the nipple core.
The assistant inserts a 3rd endoscopic grasper through the remained port and take nipple core out and send it to a pathologist for frozen biopsy.

Procedure	Details
14. Flap dissection toward the medial side of the breast	Proceed with flap dissection to the medial direction. Your sight will be obscured by the breast parenchyma because of the dome shape of the breast parenchyma. At that point, it is time to turn the camera 30° downward. When all the ink injection sites of the borders have been identified, prepare the separation of the borders.

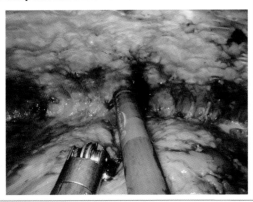

Precautions	Checklist
When carrying out the NAC dissection, you will see the yellow subcutaneous fat at the end of the fibrotic tissue of the NAC. This means you have passed the NAC.	☐ Has the NAC been identified? ☐ Is the NAC being pulled upward by an assistant? ☐ When dissecting the subareolar tissue, has the yellow subcutaneous fat on inner side been identified? ☐ Has enough of the nipple core been obtained for frozen biopsy? ☐ Has the assistant delivered the nipple core safely? ☐ Is the frozen biopsy of the nipple margin negative?
	☐ Have you changed the position of the camera with 30° downward when your sight was obscured by the breast parenchyma? ☐ Have all the borders been identified?

Procedure	Details
15. Detachment of the breast parenchyma	Dissect the borders of the breast using the left robotic arm for the traction of the breast. Starting from the free border of the inferior pole, separate the breast parenchyma in the infero–medial area to a medial and superior direction or starting from the free border of the superior pole, separate the breast parenchyma in the supero–medial area to a medial and inferior direction. When the breast parenchyma is completely separated from the borders, switch the camera back into 30° upward position. Check bleeding and the flap conditions, and release docking.
16. Specimen removal	Remove specimen via the incision site. Observe specimen and check the location of the tumor. Make sure that surgical margins are grossly intact.
17. Bleeder ligation and irrigation	After undocking, carry out hemostasis and irrigation. Measure the weight of the removed breast.
18. Reconstruction	

Precautions	Checklist
	☐ Is the breast parenchyma tractioned properly? ☐ Has the breast parenchyma been completely separated? ☐ Is there any bleeding in the operative field? ☐ Are there any injuries or bleeding from the skin flap?
If the specimen is too large to come out, remove the port and then, extend the incision length to retrieve.	☐ Is the specimen being retrieved safely? ☐ If the incision has been extended, has the final incision size been documented? ☐ Has there been anything left behind at the surgical site such as surgical equipment or foreign bodies? ☐ Are the anterior (superficial), superior, inferior, medial, lateral and posterior (basal) margins of the specimen grossly intact? ☐ If the surgical margins seem too close, has the frozen biopsy been carried out if possible?
	☐ Was the hemostasis successful? ☐ Have all significant details regarding the surgery been confirmed and documented? ☐ Has the weight of the specimen been measured?

INDEX